Praise for

JAPANESE WOMEN DON'T GET OLD OR FAT

"Moriyama walks readers through creating a 'Tokyo kitchen' in their own home—rice cooker and wok are optional—and intersperses her argument for Japanese culinary supremacy with recipes.... The result: a delicious way to stay healthy."
—*Washington Post*

"For weight loss, I recommend *Japanese Women Don't Get Old or Fat: Secrets of My Mother's Tokyo Kitchen*, by Naomi Moriyama and William Doyle. One-upping a certain French woman who boasted about staying thin, Moriyama reveals seven secrets of how Japanese women avoid adding pounds and prolong their life." —goodhousekeeping.com

"Thanks to Moriyama and Doyle, readers can learn from an insider raised in Japan who has lived in America for quite a while. Readers will learn the secrets of Japanese cooking [and] a more active lifestyle...even the most hesitant readers will find their passion for the wonderful taste and aroma of Japanese dishes irresistible and will be tempted to try some."
—*Cleveland Plain Dealer*

"Just about all the recipes come by way of Moriyama's mother, Chizuko, whom Moriyama describes as a master of 'Japan's greatest food secret of all: home cooking.' Chizuko's motto is 'I use ingredients from the mountains, the oceans and the earth.' If that isn't the Zen of cooking, what is? So pass the bonito flakes. I'll skip the Camembert, thanks."
—*AARP Magazine* online

"It's well known that Japanese women have the lowest obesity rate in the industrialized world (3%) and the highest life expectancy (85 years), and that their cuisine is based on simplicity. Tokyo native Moriyama puts a human face on this phenomenon, that of her mother, Chizuko, in this well-organized, persuasive introduction to a non-Western everyday cooking plan." —*Publishers Weekly*

Japanese Women
Don't Get Old or Fat

SECRETS OF MY MOTHER'S TOKYO KITCHEN

Naomi Moriyama

and William Doyle

DELTA TRADE PAPERBACK

JAPANESE WOMEN DON'T GET OLD OR FAT
A Delta Book

PUBLISHING HISTORY
Delacorte Press hardcover edition published November 2005
Delta Trade Paperback edition / January 2007

Published by
Bantam Dell
A Division of Random House, Inc.
New York, New York

Family crests from *Snow, Wave, Pine: Traditional Patterns in Japanese Design,*
photographs by Sadao Hibi, text by Motoji Niwa, translated by Jay W. Thomas
Published by Kodansha International Ltd., 2001
Courtesy of Kodansha International Ltd.

Book design by Glen Edelstein

Library of Congress Catalog Card Number: 2005053795

Delta is a registered trademark of Random House, Inc., and the colophon is a trademark of Random House, Inc.

ISBN 978-0-385-33998-8

Printed in the United States of America
Published simultaneously in Canada

www.bantamdell.com

11

To our families, especially our parents:
Chizuko, Shigeo, Marilou, and Bill

Contents

Introduction

I just want to get healthy.
I want to take better care of myself.
I would like to start eating healthier. I don't want all that pasta.
I would like to start eating Japanese food.

—Bill Murray as Bob Harris,
in Sofia Coppola's *Lost in Translation*

THERE IS A LAND where women live longer than everyone else on Earth.

It is a place where obesity is the lowest in the developed world.

Where forty-year-old women look like they are twenty.

It is a land where women enjoy some of the world's most delicious food, yet they have *obesity rates of only 3 percent*—less than one third that of French women . . . and less than one tenth that of American women.

It is a country of women obsessed with enjoying life—and mastering the art of healthy eating. It is a highly industrialized nation that is the second-largest economic power in the world.

The country is Japan.

And something incredible is happening there.

JAPAN AND THE GLOBAL OBESITY EPIDEMIC

Right now, the world is suffering an obesity crisis that is afflicting hundreds of millions of people.

In 2004, the World Health Organization (WHO) declared a "global obesity epidemic," with more than 1 billion adults overweight—and at least 300 million of them obese, with obesity defined as having a body mass index, or BMI, of over 30. Obesity, announced the WHO, "is a major contributor to the global burden of chronic disease and disability."

The WHO reports that the obesity epidemic is rapidly spreading beyond the United States and Western Europe into Eastern Europe, Latin America, the Middle East, and the developing world. "It's universal," said Neville Rigby, policy director of the WHO's International Obesity Task Force. "It has become a fully global epidemic, indeed, a pandemic."

There is scientific debate over the exact number of deaths attributable each year to obesity, but there is little dispute that a public health crisis is under way.

The news is alarming, and it's getting worse:

- A striking 34 percent of adult American women are obese. More than 20 percent of American men, and English and German men and women, are obese.

- Obesity in French women and men climbed from approximately 8 percent in 1997 to 11 percent in 2003, an increase of almost 40 percent.

- The U.S. National Institutes of Health estimates that obesity and overweight cost the nation an estimated $117 billion in direct medical costs and indirect costs, such as lost wages due to illness. This is more than *double* the current federal budget for homeland security.

- In a June 2, 2005 press briefing, Dr. Julie Louise Gerberding, director of the U.S. Centers for Disease Control and Prevention, linked obesity to an increased risk of hypertension, diabetes, renal failure, colon cancer, postmenopausal breast cancer, gallbladder cancer, uterine cancer, arthritis, sleep disturbances and breathing problems, as well as to problems with childbearing and premature birth.

- The state of California alone estimates its obesity-related costs at $21.7 billion a year, leading its health and human services secretary to declare in 2005 that "the obesity epidemic is more than a public health crisis, it is an economic crisis."

- Obesity in U.S. children has tripled in the last quarter century. "It boggles my mind," said Dr. William Klish, head of the department of medicine at Texas Children's Hospital. "When

I started in the 1960s and early '70s," he told the Associated Press in early 2005, "we never ever saw a case of type 2 diabetes, adult-onset diabetes, in children. Now, we're making the diagnosis routinely."

- In Australia, surgeons are struggling to cope with the demand for lap-band stomach operations for obese children. "I think epidemic's almost too polite a word," Dr. George Fielding told the Royal Australasian College of Surgeons conference in 2005. He prefers to call it a plague. Children of twelve, thirteen, and fourteen are "all getting the diseases their grandparents have," he said, "they're getting diabetes, high blood pressure, sleep apnea, and heart disease at rates that would be unbelievable ten years ago."

- The aircraft manufacturer Boeing is reengineering its designs to accommodate heavier passengers and resulting higher fuel costs. The new Boeing 7E7 aircraft, due in 2008, will feature wider aisles and seats and new structural material designed, in the words of a Boeing spokesperson, to "counteract the increasing weight of passengers."

But in the midst of this global obesity crisis, the nation of Japan has managed to become, by several key criteria, the healthiest nation in the world.

Japanese have the lowest obesity rates in the developed world.

Obesity is defined as a body mass index (BMI) of 30 or higher. The following table shows the percentage of obese adults in various developed nations.

PERCENTAGE OF ADULTS WHO ARE OBESE

	Men	Women
Greece	27	38
United States	28	34
England	22	23
Germany	22	23
Australia	19	22
Canada	16	14
France	11	11
Italy	9	10
Japan	3	3

Japanese women are the world champions of longevity.

Japan has become the Land of Immortal Women. According to the Associated Press, in 2004, "Japanese women set a new record for the world's longest life expectancy, retaining the title for the nineteenth straight year." *The Economist* recently proclaimed that "the life expectancy of Japanese men and women has been the highest in the world for a decade and is continuing to rise." Have a look at the World Health Organization's latest figures:

LIFE EXPECTANCY AT BIRTH

(IN YEARS)

	Women	Men	Both Sexes
Japan	85	78	82
Italy	84	78	81
Australia, Sweden, Switzerland	83	78	81
France	84	76	80
Spain	83	76	80
Canada, Iceland, Israel, Singapore	82	78	80
New Zealand, Norway	82	77	79
Austria, Germany, Luxembourg	82	76	79
Belgium, Finland	82	75	79
Greece, Malta, Netherlands, United Kingdom	81	76	79
Cyprus, Ireland	81	76	78
United States	80	75	77

**Japanese are not just living longest,
they're living healthiest.**

According to a recent article in the *Washington Post*, "Japanese are not only the longest-lived but statistically the healthiest seniors in the world. The typical Japanese senior now enjoys at least seventy-five years of relative good health." According to the WHO's latest "healthy life expectancy" figures, which, in contrast to the life expectancy figures above, estimate the average number of *healthy, disability-free* years a group will live:

- Japanese women expect the most years of *healthy life expectancy* at birth among all men or women in the world's 192 nations: 77.7 years of good health.
- Japanese men enjoy the most years of healthy life expectancy among all men in the world's 192 nations.
- Japanese people have the most years of healthy longevity among all nations, beating the French and Germans by three years, the British by four years, and the Americans, who rank twenty-third in the world, by almost six years.

Japanese are achieving this while actually spending less on health care.

HEALTH CARE SPENDING PER PERSON PER YEAR
(IN U.S. DOLLARS)

United States	5,707
Germany	3,849
France	3,601
United Kingdom	3,224
Japan	2,839

All this leads up to an intriguing question, which could be called the Japanese Paradox: How can the world's most food-obsessed nation have the lowest obesity rates in the industrialized world—and the best longevity on Earth?

Experts point to a number of factors, including lifestyle and strong social and spiritual ties. And many experts agree that

Take a stroll through Tokyo, or any other Japanese city for that matter, and you'll almost immediately notice that the Japanese are an awesomely healthy-looking race of people. . . . The Japanese also have lower rates of stroke, breast cancer and prostate cancer. And on a more superficial level, they tend to look, on average, at least ten years younger. Their eyes are bright, their skin glows and their hair is glossy.

—Kelly Baker, *journalist*

one other aspect of the Japanese way of life makes a big difference: diet. "I think that the Asian diet is probably the world's healthiest," says Dr. Dean Ornish, director of the Preventive Medicine Research Institute in California. "The diet that we use that we found can reverse prostate cancer is really based on the Asian diet. Whether you call it a Japanese diet or a Chinese diet—predominantly fruits, vegetables, whole grains, legumes, soy products in their natural form, and for people who are trying to prevent heart disease, a little bit of fish, more as a condiment than as a main course."

JAPANESE HOME COOKING

A good part of the answer to the Japanese Paradox, in fact, lies inside a Tokyo kitchen, in the magic of Japanese home cooking, in the kind of food prepared by my mother—and by millions of other Japanese mothers. And that is what I want to tell you about in this book.

However, this is not a diet book.

And it's not a book about making sushi.

My mother doesn't make sushi that often, and I don't make it at all. I love eating sushi, but I leave sushi making to the experts.

In other words, this is not a book about Japanese restaurant food.

This book is an introduction to a whole new way of eating at home—Japanese home-style cooking. There is some overlap with Japanese restaurant cuisine, but a lot of what Japanese eat every day with their families is different, and easier to make, than what you may expect.

This is a book about discovering the joy and fun of everyday Japanese home-style cooking.

And this is a book that explores the opinions of a number of the world's experts on longevity and obesity, who offer their insights on the subject of how Japanese food habits may be contributing to the extraordinary good health of the Japanese people.

Finally, this is a book that will show you how to make some of the classic dishes that Japanese women make for their own families. It will explain the basics, and in the chapter called How to Start Your Tokyo Kitchen, I will describe the basic ingredients you need to make them. (Remember that if you see ingredients on a recipe list that you don't recognize, the information on what they are and where to find them is close at hand.)

I think you too can start to make Japanese home-cooked dishes—and I think you're going to be great at it.

And when you do, I'm pretty sure of one thing.

You're going to feel fantastic.

CHAPTER I

My Mother's Tokyo Kitchen

The people assemble in joy;
Food and drink is abundant.
For all generations without end,
Day by day ever more flourishing,
Until myriads of years hence
The pleasure will not cease.

—Ancient Japanese blessing

MY MOTHER, CHIZUKO, sends me e-mails from Tokyo all the time.

She sends them from her mobile phone—when she's in the kitchen or the grocery store, when she's on line to buy tickets to a show, or when she's waiting for a train in a Tokyo subway station.

She wants to know how my husband, Billy, and I are doing, when we're coming over to visit—and what we're eating.

To help us write this book, she's been sending us her recipes and food tips by e-mail and via fax, sometimes writing little diagrams of vegetables like mountain potatoes. She is a self-taught natural master of Japanese home cooking who never refers to a cookbook. "It's all in my brain," she explains.

Like many mothers in Japan and around the world, my mother has always been devoted to giving her family the most healthy and delicious food she can find, as a way of showing her love for them.

I see her cooking not just as a sign of love but also as the perfect symbol of why Japanese women are living longer and healthier than everyone else on Earth, and why they (and their husbands) have the lowest obesity rates in the developed world.

My husband and I both have stories to tell that bring those statistics to life.

I'll start with Billy's story, which began several years ago, when we stayed at my parents' apartment in Tokyo for a week and experienced—for the first time, in Billy's case—a total immersion in my mother's home cooking. I had been back to Tokyo many times over the years, both on business and to visit my family, but when I was there I usually stayed at hotels like the Park Hyatt (the setting of Sofia Coppola's *Lost in Translation*). This time, we chose not to stay in a hotel because my parents insisted on our being with them.

For me, that week in my mother's Tokyo kitchen was a delicious reawakening to the tastes and aromas of my youth, of the years before I moved to New York at the age of twenty-seven. For Billy, it was a completely new experience.

Billy had been to Tokyo with me once before, but on that trip we had separate business meetings in different parts of town, we stayed in a Western-style hotel, and I was too busy to introduce him to the pleasures of Tokyo food, which was completely foreign and intimidating to him.

Billy wandered the streets of Tokyo in a state of hungry confusion.

He looked in shop windows and stared at noodle bowls and bento boxes—and he was clueless. He had no idea what or how to order. The food looked strange and the menus were incomprehensible.

Food was everywhere—but to him it all seemed out of reach.

So he made a beeline for McDonald's, and chowed down on Big Macs, shakes, and fries almost every day, he confessed later.

At the end of four days in Tokyo, he felt lousy and was five pounds fatter.

But during his next trip to Tokyo, after a week of eating only the dishes that emerged from my mother's Tokyo kitchen, Billy had fallen madly in love with Japanese home-cooked food. When we went back to New York, he continued eating Japanese-style food almost exclusively.

For both of us, that week in Tokyo ignited a new passion for the joys of Japanese home cooking.

Before that trip, we relied heavily on takeout, frozen dinners, and eating out, just like other New York workaholics. To me, "cooking" meant buying prewashed salad mix from a supermarket, putting it in a pretty bowl, and serving it with a premium-priced dressing. My repertory was otherwise limited to cooking dry pasta in boiling water, sautéing broccoli and tomatoes, and mixing them with bottled marinara sauce.

Preparing a meal from scratch was rare. Who had the

energy? By the time I left my office in the evening, I was exhausted and left with no brainpower to think about a menu, let alone the energy to wash and chop vegetables.

But after that week at my parents' house, Billy and I started to prepare Japanese-style meals at home more and more often, especially after Billy learned to make rice like a professional and even cook miso soup for breakfast. We quickly realized that we could re-create my mother's Tokyo kitchen at our apartment in New York.

I began going to local Japanese grocery stores for tofu, seasoning products like soy sauce, rice vinegar, and miso, and the local supermarkets and farmers market for fresh vegetables, meat, and fish. The more I visited Japanese grocery stores, the more I remembered the kind of dishes I used to eat when I lived with my parents, dishes like grilled fish and simmered root vegetables.

And the most surprising thing was that the more Japanese home cooking we ate, the leaner, more energetic, and more productive we became, while at the same time feeling completely satisfied after every meal. Part of the reason for writing this book was simply to collect Chizuko's recipes and techniques so we could tape them to our own refrigerator.

In 2004 we began researching the subject in depth, and discovered a wide range of scientific and journalistic evidence suggesting the health benefits of traditional Japanese home cooking and ingredients and lifestyle habits. This helped explain to us why we felt so much better after we started cooking the way my mother does.

But I want to reassure you that this is not a cuisine you should find intimidating, even though aspects of it are very different from what you may be used to. Japanese food, in many ways, has already become American food.

Across the nation, Americans have fallen in love with Japanese restaurants and take-out sushi. In Houston alone there are more than a hundred Japanese eateries. Japanese foods and ingredients like edamame, ponzu, wasabi, yuzu, and miso have become standard items in non-Japanese restaurant kitchens. Now it's time to discover Japan's greatest food secret of all: home cooking.

———

I left the comfort of my mother's Tokyo kitchen twice. The first time was when I went away to college; the second was when I moved to New York. But twice I returned to it, each time very glad that I did. And now that I've re-created a Tokyo kitchen in my own home, I'll never leave again, at least not for long.

DREAMING OF FOOD UTOPIA

I grew up in Japan, in a city that is the Food Utopia of Planet Earth—Tokyo.

As I sit in my office in New York City, I close my eyes . . . *and I can taste it.*

I take a deep breath.
I am in my mother's Tokyo kitchen.

I am drenched in a narcotic mixture of the subtle, sweet, and earthy fragrances I've been tasting since I was a little girl.

The kitchen smells like the earth, the sea, and the mountains—*it smells like life.*

My mother, a short, black-haired, ultra-high-energy Japanese woman, is making our family dinner with the speed of a panther, the confidence of Martha Stewart, and the precision of a NASA scientist.

Green tea is brewing in an earthenware pot.

Fresh green and yellow vegetables are simmering in dashi, a clear broth made from bonito flakes, kelp, and mushrooms. Fluffy rice is plumping up in the rice cooker, steaming out a rich nutty flavor.

My mother grills small slices of fish with a light touch of lemon and canola oil, then polishes little squares of tofu with a brown sauce before lining up bowls of simmering miso soup made from scratch. They look like jewel boxes.

Through the window of my parent's little penthouse apartment, the vast megapolis of Tokyo stretches out to near infinity, with Mt. Fuji capping the western horizon. The wind is shooting ribbon clouds of snow off the peak. My father, Shigeo, sits in his easy chair, admiring the mountain intently through his field glasses.

On the sofa nearby is my husband, a native New Yorker who hardly ever ate Japanese food until several years ago, when he came to my parents' house for a week and ate my mother's Japanese cooking three times a day, every day (not that he had a choice!).

He was startled to discover that it was, in his words, "the most amazingly delicious, energy-boosting food I ever tasted" and he soon began eating nothing else, even in New York.

My mom changed the way Billy eats, weighs, and feels, forever.

Before going to Tokyo, he weighed nearly 220 pounds.

Today, he holds steady around 185. He mostly eats Japanese-style food.

He went from a size 42 waist to a size 36.

He traveled through three different body types, starting with "obese" (he had a body mass index of 30), progressing to "overweight" (a BMI of 28), and on to where he is today—"normal" (a BMI just below 25).

I've spent half my life in Japan and most of the other half in America. I love both countries and I have eaten at some of their finest restaurants: Nobu, the Four Seasons, and Sushi Yasuda in New York, the New York Grill in Tokyo, and Takeshigero in Kyoto.

But my mother's Tokyo kitchen is my favorite place to eat on Earth, and I come here as often as I can, usually several times a year.

As I picture myself hovering over my mother, trying to learn all her cooking secrets, my reverie is suddenly broken by the image of her chasing me out of the kitchen and calling everyone to the table by announcing, *"Gohan desu yo!"* This means "rice is ready," which, since every meal in Japan has rice, means "the meal is ready."

What comes out of my mother's kitchen is not complicated sushi or elaborate, formal kaiseki dishes. This is good old-fashioned, hard-core everyday Japanese mom's cooking.

It's what tens of millions of Japanese mothers and wives serve their families every day. It is the food my mother fed me

as a little girl, as a high school student, and even as a young executive trainee in my first office job in Tokyo, when she would
sometimes chase down the street after me with a piece of toast
if I rushed out of the apartment without eating.

My mom's dishes are a mixture of traditional Japanese home
cooking and her own creative improvisations. They include
Western-style dishes like fried eggs, pasta, salads, and soups, usually reconfigured to suit her taste and her healthy style of cooking.
They always incorporate ingredients that are super-fresh.

My mom's Tokyo kitchen is tiny, about six by twelve feet. It
is jam-packed and piled high with cooking utensils, plates, and
seasoning stuff. She has virtually no counter space.

When my good friend Susan came to Tokyo from New
York to visit for a couple of days on the way to Hong Kong, she
witnessed my mom whip up a few fantastic dishes out of thin
air, in a scene right out of "The Sorcerer's Apprentice." Susan
still talks about it ten years later.

THE FRESHNESS MANTRA

When I was growing up, we rarely ate out or brought takeout
foods home. My mom said she could do it better and cheaper.
She did—and she still does.

She shops for ingredients from a variety of places—from local supermarkets, department store food courts, downtown
Tokyo specialty stores, and the Tsukiji fish market. Every day
she goes to local stores for fresh fish, meat, and vegetables, and
back when there was a family-owned tofu store nearby that
made fresh tofu on the premises, she even bought her tofu
fresh. She often does not decide what dishes to make before she

Naomi's mother's Tokyo kitchen was an out-of-body experience.

First was its size. No bigger than a modest-size walk-in closet, it yielded a cornucopia of preciously and precisely stacked ingredients and cooking accoutrements. Trying to open a drawer or cupboard put my clandestine 4 A.M. jet-lagged forays at risk. I feared that I could suffer a mighty burial by the kitchen's contents at any moment.

Second was what came out of the kitchen. I have never in my adult life indulged, tried and enjoyed the kind of epicurean delights placed in front of me. I hate fish, but not from Naomi's mother's Tokyo kitchen. I ate cooked pumpkin in bewilderment, wondering where in that kitchen the pumpkin could have been. I ate green leaf-like mountains of something, only to realize that seaweed could taste good.

Third and most significant of all, was the mistress of this place (Chizuko Moriyama). Barely five feet, always smiling, nodding and bowing to me (due to a significant language barrier), she made me *want* to eat all of her food.

I hope to return someday, only en famille. I am hopeful she will get my three boys to eat fish.

—Susan D. Plagemann, Vice President, Publisher, *Marie Claire* magazine, and visitor to my mother's Tokyo kitchen

goes grocery shopping. Only after she's looked over the market's offerings and seen what looks fresh and fabulous that day does she devise her menu plan. For perishables, "freshness" is a Tokyo kitchen mantra. Whether it is fish, fruits, vegetables, or herbs, if it is in season and available fresh, that's what Japanese women buy. If it's not fresh, they stay away.

For a while, when our family lived in Kawasaki, a city next to Tokyo where my father had a job as an engineer at a chemical company, we even grew some vegetables next to our flower beds. We had a little garden patch, planted with corn, parsley, tomatoes, and eggplant, and we had a fig tree growing outside the kitchen windows, so close that we could almost reach out and pick the fruit without even going outside.

We also had chickens. We were the only family in the neighborhood with chickens running around the backyard! Actually, they were a bantam mini-chicken creature of the type known as "chabo," which have been kept as house pets in Japan ever since the early days of Edo (old Tokyo), when someone started importing them from what is now Vietnam. The chabo used to dig little holes in our garden with their feet, and sit in them among the flower bushes, so still they looked like they were meditating. Every morning my sister and I would go out to gather the eggs, which were sometimes so newly laid that they were warm to the touch, and my mom would cook them for us. She adored those little chabo chickens. Although I didn't have any particular feeling for them at the time, looking back I realize that the chabo kept us connected to nature in the midst of the steel plants, oil refineries, and factories that were not far away. The eggs they laid and the fruits and vegetables we grew reflected my mother's dedication to cooking with the freshest possible ingredients.

My mom was probably the first Japanese housewife to own an imported General Electric refrigerator. It was the second largest piece of furniture—after the piano—in our apartment. It was too big for a Japanese-size kitchen, so it had to sit outside, sort of on the edge of our dining room. But cooking and having fresh ingredients were such passions of hers that she had to have that refrigerator, outsize as it was.

A LOVE-PACKED LUNCH BOX

From ages twelve to eighteen, my younger sister, Miki, and I went to an all-girls private school in Kawasaki.

On the first day of school all the mothers and daughters were seated in the auditorium and a teacher at the podium made an orientation speech:

> We request that every mother make lunch for your daughter every day.
>
> Our main theme at this school is to help our students learn to be giving and loving. One of the ways your daughter learns this is from your love-packed lunch box.
>
> We understand that there might be times when a mother has an emergency and cannot prepare lunch. We provide a sandwich and lunch box stand at school, but it is not for every day. It is for only occasional uses when it cannot be avoided.

My mother took this speech very seriously.

For years, she woke up at 6 A.M. and cooked small portions of fish, veggies, eggs, and meat for us, sliced them up, and packed them neatly and elegantly along with a sheet of nori seaweed over a bed of rice in a small airtight Tupperware lunch box.

She wrapped up the lunch in a cloth napkin with my name and flowers embroidered in a corner. She made these napkins too.

Every day the lunch box contained different side dishes, sandwiches, or rice balls. She made every lunch box with total dedication and passion.

One day, I untied the napkin, opened the plastic wrap, and started eating a sandwich. I was surprised to find a sheet of nori seaweed on top of the ham and cheese.

My schoolmates and I were accustomed to British-style sandwiches, with lettuce, thinly sliced cucumbers, tomatoes, ham, and cheese. Nori seaweed was something we ate in Japanese dishes, never in a sandwich. As a self-conscious teenager, I was awfully embarrassed to be seen eating that seaweed in front of my schoolmates.

I went home and said to my mother, "Nobody puts seaweed in a sandwich!"

She said, "Well, seaweed is good for you, but I will try not to do it again."

Today I realize I was too young to appreciate her creativity.

Mom's Carrot-Tofu Dish

SERVES 4

Loaded with fragrant toasted and ground sesame seeds, this carrot-tofu mixture is one of my favorite dishes. It's my mother's unique creation and was a star side dish in my lunch box at high school. While I often eat it hot with freshly cooked rice, it tastes wonderful when cold, especially on toasted whole grain bread. Delicious!

> Two 3-x-5-inch rectangles usu-age tofu (thin-fried tofu)
> 2 tablespoons rice vinegar
> 2 teaspoons granulated sugar
> 2 teaspoons sake
> 2 teaspoons reduced-sodium soy sauce
> 1 teaspoon salt
> 1 tablespoon canola oil or rice bran oil
> 6 cups matchsticks of carrot (from about 5 medium carrots)
> 1/3 cup toasted and ground white sesame seeds (page 111)
> 2 teaspoons toasted sesame oil

1. Bring a small saucepan of water to a boil. Add the usu-age tofu and gently simmer over medium heat, turning occasionally, for 1 minute; drain (this will remove excess oil). Cut the usu-age tofu diagonally in half and slice each half into thin strips.

2. Combine the vinegar, sugar, sake, soy, and salt in a small bowl. Stir until the sugar has dissolved.

3. Heat the oil in a large skillet over high heat. Add the carrots and usu-age tofu strips and sauté until the carrots are crisp-tender, about 3 minutes. Reduce the heat to medium-low and add the soy mixture. Cook the carrots and tofu for 2 more minutes, or until tender (but not too soft). Turn off the heat, stir in the sesame seeds, and drizzle with the toasted sesame oil.

4. Transfer to a small serving dish.

WELCOME TO JAPAN, THE WORLD'S MOST FOOD-OBSESSED NATION

Japan is a nation of ardent epicures. And Japanese women are the high priestesses of Food Utopia.

The Italians are passionate about food, of course, as are the French, and the Americans, and the Spanish, and the Chinese, and the people of practically every other nation.

But you have to walk the streets of Japan yourself to actually believe how all-consuming Japan's food obsession is. Japan may be only the second largest economy, but it is literally the world's Food Utopia.

When I say "obsession," I don't mean an irrational, weird fixation. I mean a true love and devotion to delicious, healthy food. It is a magnificent obsession.

To most Americans, Japanese food means sushi. Sushi is fantastic, and it's one of Japan's favorite foods, but it's only one of many. All across Japan, you can find a myriad of fabulous food.

It's not that we're snobby about it (although we can be downright finicky), it's just that somehow Japanese have come to expect culinary excellence as almost a birthright.

For example, take an escalator down to the basement of any big Japanese department store, like Isetan, Mitsukoshi, or Takashimaya: you will be transported into a vast, teeming paradise of food, its landscapes bedecked with elegant gourmet dishes, exquisite take-out lunch boxes, and row after row of glass display cases filled with chocolate truffles, cookies, and pastries next to traditional Japanese confectionary, all of it freshly made.

Almost all the cookies are tiny bite-size morsels (1 inch square or smaller), never like those typical gigantic American cookies that often reach a diameter of 4 to 5 inches. Modestly sweetened but very flavorful, Japanese cookies are likely to come individually wrapped, in a bag or can, encouraging you to enjoy just one or two cookies at a time and save the rest for later.

Everywhere you look, you see the highest-quality food ingredients, the finest, freshest produce, and the most beautifully packaged gourmet meals to go.

These Tokyo take-out foods are not just Japanese, but Italian, Chinese, French, and Indian, since food in Japan has been a global affair for many centuries. The Chinese influence on Japanese food dates back well over a thousand years. Tempura, which we think of as quintessentially Japanese, was inspired by the dishes of visiting Portuguese traders in the 1500s. And after Japan opened up to the West in the late nineteenth century, all kinds of international products took off: meat, curry, pork, and bread, and eventually coffee, French food, pizza, and pastries.

Chocolate is another food we learned about from the West. And we value it very highly. One elegant Tokyo department store now offers shoppers their own accounts in a Chocolate Bank—you buy an amount of gourmet chocolate, the store keeps it in its temperature-controlled chocolate vault, and you stop in to make a withdrawal any time you want.

Even in this ultramodern high-tech city, with all its sophisticated foreign influences, the old traditional Japan is never too far away. Billy and I discovered this when we rented an apartment in the Aoyama district of Tokyo last summer. Close to midnight one night we heard a man's voice singing *"Gy— oooo—za, gy—oooo—za!"* A guy in a minivan filled with hot dumplings was slowly wandering through the back streets, offering gyoza dumplings as a late-night snack. He was singing the tune in the same melody passed down from generation to generation by the Tokyo sweet potato vendors who still peddle their wares in certain neighborhoods of Tokyo.

Food is everywhere in Japan, all the time, and the quality and freshness standards are ruthlessly high—higher, I think, than anywhere else on the planet. It's what Japanese women demand and what businesses and restaurants have to deliver.

Little shops offering mouthwatering home-style noodle dishes are to be found on almost every downtown street. The cities of Japan are overflowing with fantastic restaurants featuring foods from around the world. Some of the best French restaurants outside France are in Japan. TV networks are flooded with food programs. In Japan, gourmet food is not just for the wealthy, it's for everyone.

Japanese supermarkets are cathedrals of freshness. Food is not only dated, *it's timed*—Japanese women buy fish, meat, vegetables, or prepared meals that are timed by the half hour they were packed that day. There is relatively little frozen and canned food in Japanese cooking—the emphasis is on food that is *shun*, or in season. Even the inexpensive take-out sandwiches and rice balls at convenience stores are super-fresh and delicious.

According to writer Peggy Orenstein, who described a Tokyo culinary sojourn in an article she wrote for *Health* magazine, Japan is proof that fast food can be good food.

"On the go, I slurped buckwheat noodles in a clear, tasty

broth at a soba-noodle stand," Orenstein recalled. "One day, I tailed a group of young office workers at lunchtime and discovered that local 7-Elevens have surprisingly decent chow. I'm serious. I bought a bento box of grilled salmon; two seaweed-wrapped rice balls; tamago (omelette); and a salad of spinach, grated carrots, and yam noodles with sesame sauce."

Global retail giant Wal-Mart has invested in Japanese supermarket chain Seiyu so it could learn Japanese secrets of food distribution and freshness.

Japanese are not food saints in every respect: many young Japanese wolf down fast food from places like McDonald's, and there's been a recent alarming spike in obesity among those Japanese who don't exercise enough and adopt less healthy Western-style eating habits.

Furthermore, there is way too much salt in the Japanese diet—in foods like salted dried fish, pickled vegetables, and soy sauce. Experts speculate that excessive sodium in the Japanese diet may contribute to high blood pressure, stroke, and stomach cancer. So I always suggest you look for lower-sodium options for things like soy sauce and miso.

Another problem: there is very strong social pressure for women in Japan to be slim, since it's a society that has never gotten used to the idea of people being overweight. Unfortunately, this has led some young women to fall victim to eating disorders and extreme thinness. As in many developed countries, eating disorders like anorexia are on the rise.

Besides these food-related problems, Japanese still smoke too much. The rates of lung cancer and bronchial diseases are unacceptably high, as are alcohol-related ailments.

An unbelievable 50 percent of Japanese men still smoke, the worst rate in the entire industrialized world. (This compares with 10 percent of Japanese women.)

Yet on balance, and compared to the rest of the world, an extraordinary number of Japanese live a very healthy lifestyle—in large part because of what they eat.

And the proof is that something incredible is happening in this food-crazed land—the women and men are living longer than everyone else on Earth, and you will hardly ever see any obese people in Japan. At the same time, very few people in Japan go hungry.

How do the Japanese do it?
One reason is that they eat much, much differently than people in the West.

CHAPTER 2

In a Japanese Tangerine Forest

A father's favor overtops the mountains;
A mother's kindness is deeper than the sea.

—Traditional Japanese proverb

I CLOSE MY EYES.

I am five years old.
I am in a tangerine orchard in the mountains of rural Japan.

I've got a basket tied around my waist, and I'm filling it with ripe, juicy tangerines that I'm clipping from the trees. The landscape looks like a Vincent van Gogh painting—splashed with bright shades of orange and green paint.

I am surrounded by lush hillsides groaning with the weight of persimmons, radishes, scallions, and potatoes.

This is where I spent some of the happiest summer days of my childhood, visiting my paternal grandparents' traditional farm compound in a village named Kozaka in Mie Prefecture on the Kii peninsula. It's about two hours southwest of Tokyo via a bullet train (or *shinkansen*) and a connecting local train.

The region around my grandparents' farm is known for its tangerines, for Matsuzaka beef (which some think is even tastier than Kobe beef), and for Mikimoto cultured pearls, which are today still plucked from the coastal depths by expert female divers in white swimsuits and snorkels.

It is a countryside that can inspire rhapsodic feelings in visitors, one of whom, journalist Jeremy Ferguson, described it in Canada's *Globe and Mail* as "a remarkably lovely corner of Japan, unspoiled and uncrowded . . . Coniferous jungle covers its mountains. The green fire of rice paddies fans through the lowlands. The sea coast undulates in S-curves, punctuated with oyster beds and islands so pleasing to behold, they qualify as sculpture." The sunsets over the tangerine forests are so beautiful, he noted, they inspire haiku poetry.

For me, this was a food playground, and an advanced education in traditional Japanese country-style eating, courtesy of my father's family, many of whom were, and still are, part-time working farmers. According to family lore, they have been farming on this spot for the past three hundred years.

My grandfather, Kumezo, worked on the farm until the last years of his life. He lived to be ninety-five. My grandparents and their family grew tea, rice, barley, and wheat on the farm, plus three types of tangerines, five types of persimmons, plums, and no fewer than thirty different types of vegetables.

The farm also had milk-giving cows in a pen, and, running around the yard, chickens that provided a daily supply of eggs for the family.

Everything in this community revolved around food. The families of the village, like many in the Japanese countryside, are interconnected in a semicommunal web of cooperative farms and related businesses.

When my parents, my sister, and I went there for summer vacations, we stayed in the long, two-story, straw-roofed Moriyama family farmhouse, which accommodated up to four generations at a time. It had many rooms with tatami mat floors, and a bathroom with a tub made of stone. My grandmother, Tsune, would burn logs underneath the bathtub to heat the water. The restroom was outside, next to the cow hut.

The days began at 5 A.M. My grandmother would walk out to the cultivated hillside behind the house and pick a bushel of fresh fruit and vegetables for the family breakfast. As I men-

> The sudden freshness of Japanese cuisine captures attention as does a whisper in the midst of shouts. One detects, in presentation and in flavor, authenticity. Things are introduced and eaten in varying degrees of rawness, nothing is overcooked; one feels near the food in its natural state.
>
> —Donald Richie, A Taste of Japan

tioned earlier, Japanese home cooks are extremely concerned with freshness, and it can't get any fresher than this—we were eating food just an hour after it was harvested.

My grandmother, who lived until age ninety, was a great home cook. "Every dish she made was simple and did not require any special skills or techniques," remembers my dad. "For example, she boiled vegetables like eggplants, green peppers, onions, and burdock, and seasoned them with miso paste. She made rice-vinegared dishes with cucumbers or squash, and gave them some punch with chopped green shiso leaves."

The front door to the kitchen was always open, and neighbors and cousins would stream in and out all day long to visit, chat, and sip some green tea. On the kitchen table was a serving area that was usually filled with some healthy snacks, typically rows of rice balls on a tray. As people came and went, the rice balls disappeared one by one, until the tray was empty. As a city girl visiting from Tokyo, I watched the constant comings and goings of casual visitors with wonder and awe.

For family meals, we all sat down cross-legged on pillows on the tatami mat floor—there were no chairs, in the Japanese style. Adults had heated sake with dinner, declaring, "A bit of sake is good for your health!"

The meals were incredibly simple and fresh, and most of the food came from the family farm or the farms nearby: fluffy steaming white rice, miso soup with chopped vegetables and a whole egg, sautéed meat and steamed vegetables as a main dish, and a side dish of pickled Japanese apricots (or *umeboshi*).

Not much in the way of saturated fat, refined sugar, or processed foods to be found.

I doubt that a molecule of junk food ever dared cross the threshold of that farm.

My favorite dish was hinona: coarse dark green turnip leaves that my grandmother would lightly boil, squeeze, chop, and season with rice vinegar, soy sauce, bonito flakes, or ground white sesame seeds. It was so mouthwateringly hearty that I begged my grandmother to make it every day.

Things haven't changed too much since then. I know this because Billy and I recently went back to Kozaka. Visiting my cousin Yoshikazu, who runs the farm now, and my uncle Masao, who has a family grocery and restaurant near the village, we sat down with the extended family to participate in a communal meal.

That night's dinner was shabu shabu, a dish in which thin strips of beef and cut up pieces of fresh vegetables are quickly cooked in a single sizzling pot of broth. ("Shabu shabu," as you may know, is the sound the beef makes when you swish it around.) During the meal, we looked around at all my cousins and aunts and uncles, young and old, most of them sporting flaming red apple cheeks and jet-black hair that almost glistened. Everyone looked young, lean, and radiant with positive energy.

If the way they look is any indication, I thought, these people must be eating the healthiest diet on earth.

Spinach with Bonito Flakes

SERVES 4

My grandmother Tsune Moriyama made this heartily delicious, energy-boosting salad with hinona turnip leaves. In lieu of fresh hinona, I substitute spinach. You can also use greens like kale, collard, or beet leaves instead of the spinach.

1 pound of spinach, roots and coarse
　　bottom of stems removed
2 tablespoons dashi (page 52)
1 1/2 teaspoons reduced-sodium soy sauce
1 teaspoon rice vinegar
1/2 teaspoon granulated sugar
Pinch of salt
1/4 cup small bonito flakes

1. Place the spinach in a large bowl filled with water and swish the leaves around to rinse off any grit, but do not allow the bunch to separate, because you want all the leaves to remain at the top of the bunch, the stems at the bottom. If necessary, rinse two or more times in fresh water until all the dirt is gone.

2. Bring a large saucepan of water to a boil. Carefully add the spinach and cook over medium-high heat for 30 seconds, continuing to keep the bunch of spinach intact. Drain and refresh under cold water. Gently squeeze the spinach to release excess

water. After squeezing, you should have a 1- to 2-inch-thick log of spinach that is probably about 6 inches long.

3. Blend together the dashi, soy, rice vinegar, sugar, and a generous pinch of salt in a small bowl until the sugar dissolves.

4. Cut spinach leaves and stems into 1-inch chunks and squeeze out any excess water.

5. To serve, place the chunks on their ends in a medium-size serving bowl, pour the soy-vinegar mixture over them, and garnish with the bonito flakes.

CHAPTER 3

Seven Secrets from My Mother's Tokyo Kitchen

I use ingredients from the mountains, the oceans, and the earth.

—Chizuko Moriyama

LET'S GET RIGHT to the heart of what happens inside my mother's Tokyo kitchen, and inside the kitchens of tens of millions of Japanese women: the food my mother prepares has a number of qualities that make it uniquely Japanese and wonderfully healthy. The differences can be summed up in what I have called the seven secrets of Japanese home-style cooking.

SECRET 1
The Japanese diet is based on fish, soy, rice, vegetables, and fruit.

The vast majority of Japanese dishes are variations on these five simple but highly versatile themes: fish, soy, rice, vegetables and fruit.

The *classic* Japanese home-cooked meal is a piece of grilled fish, a bowl of rice, simmered vegetables, a serving of miso soup, sliced fruit for dessert, and a cup of hot green tea. In the most basic sense, a typical Japanese meal means simply a bowl of rice, a bowl of soup, and three side dishes.

Japanese consume more than twice as much fish per capita than Americans, and over ten times more soy products.

Japanese eat mountains of rice.

And Japanese are crazy about vegetables, especially fresh ones like leafy greens, daikon radish, and eggplant. A December 17, 2004, MSNBC broadcast titled "Help Ward Off Cancer with a Japanese Diet" reported: "There are many differences between Japanese and American diets that may explain why cancer incidence in Japan is far lower than in the United States. But one difference may be overlooked: the Japanese consume about five times the amount of cruciferous vegetables that Americans do." Cruciferous vegetables include cabbage, broccoli, brussels sprouts, cauliflower, kale, and watercress, and these are among the favorites in Japanese home cooking.

Another of Japan's favorite vegetables is seaweed, the nutrition-packed vegetable harvested from the sea. Kombu, nori, and wakame are all forms of seaweed. Lots more on seaweed later.

Simple and nutritious as it is, don't think that a diet based mainly on fish, soy, rice, vegetables, and fruit feels monotonous or restricted. In fact, Japanese manage to find a tremendous range of variety within these goalposts. A study of two hundred elderly Japanese women found they ate more than one hundred different foods each week, versus just thirty in a typical Western diet.

The Japanese eat less than twenty pounds of beef per year, compared with more than sixty pounds per capita in the United States. Meat is a main dish much less often than in America, and when it is served, it is sliced thin and served sparingly.

Japanese love noodles, in the form of udon and buckwheat soba, but they eat them in smaller portions than pasta-loving Americans. You can get American foods like pizza and cheeseburgers for takeout in Japan, but they're rarely eaten at home. Milk, butter, cheese, pasta, and red meat are served at home, but less often and in smaller amounts.

"When you look at it, on the surface Japan is very westernized, but westernized in a Japanese way," explains Mitsunori Murata, a nutrition expert and professor of pediatrics at Tokyo Women's Medical College. "Maybe we will eat a hamburger, but it will be Japanese-size, not American."

These eating habits explain why the Japanese diet is lower in fat (especially the animal and saturated kinds) than the American diet. The Japanese diet contains 26 percent fat, compared with 34 percent for an American diet. The Japanese diet is also lower in sugar and calories. And the fish-based diet means Japanese get higher doses of "good fats" like omega-3.

The amount of processed and refined foods consumed per capita in Japan is less than in the West, and the total amount of calories consumed by Japanese is markedly lower than in any other developed nation. The funny thing is, though, I rarely hear any Japanese complaining about how hungry they are!

DAILY CALORIE INTAKE PER PERSON

Japan	2,761
Australia	3,054
United Kingdom	3,412
Germany	3,496
Canada	3,589
France	3,654
Italy	3,671
United States	3,774

Pan-Fried Atlantic Mackerel

SERVES 4

This is an easy and delicious way to pan-fry fish after marinating it in a little sake. I also recommend an alternate method, where the fish is seasoned with pepper and dusted with flour before cooking.

Four 4-ounce fillets Atlantic mackerel
4 teaspoons sake
Pinch of salt
1 ½ tablespoons canola oil or rice bran oil
1 cup finely grated daikon radish, excess liquid
   drained off
Reduced-sodium soy sauce, to use at the table

1. Place the fish fillets in a shallow dish and season both sides with the sake and a pinch of salt.
2. Heat the oil in a large nonstick skillet over high heat. When hot, add the fish and shake the pan several times to prevent the fillets from sticking. Pan-fry the fish over medium heat for 4 minutes. Turn and fry the mackerel for 2 more minutes, or until the center of one fillet flakes when prodded with a sharp knife.
3. Transfer the fish to individual plates, and place a small amount of grated daikon next to the fillet. Let diners drizzle soy sauce over the daikon to flavor, then put the grated daikon and soy mixture onto the fish.

Variation

Place ¼ cup all-purpose flour on a large plate. Add freshly ground black pepper to the seasonings in step 1. Lightly blot the fillets with a paper towel, to soak up any excess sake, then dredge in the flour. Shake off any excess flour, and cook as described above.

SECRET 2
The Japanese eat much smaller portions, and serve them on beautiful, small-size tableware.

I was born and raised in Tokyo, but for some reason I always thought I was American as well as Japanese. For years I yearned to go to the United States, and when I was nineteen my wish came true: I received a scholarship to attend college there.

Every year, Caritas, my college in Yokohama, Japan, offered one student a two-year full scholarship for tuition and board at its sister college, Lewis University in Romeoville, Illinois. When they chose me, it seemed like the perfect ticket to the unknown alternative world I had been dreaming about—though I had only the vaguest idea of where the school was located.

My parents and I studied the U.S. map and saw that the school was in the Midwest, a place we knew nothing about, and it was somewhere not too far from Chicago. I would be the first person from either my mother's or my father's family to live in America, and this was going to be my first experience of traveling to a foreign country. I had not gone abroad even for a vacation until then.

My first day in the United States was a series of shocks.

I landed at O'Hare Airport at 6 A.M. The drive from Chicago astonished me. I had never seen such huge highways, not to mention the flat land and limitless horizon, with a sky that seemed to go on forever. No matter which direction I faced, the sky took up almost my entire field of vision.

By 7 A.M, I had arrived at school. I was escorted to the student dining room and asked what I wanted for breakfast.

"Orange juice," I said.

I was offered a very large glass of orange juice. My eyes widened in amazement. I wondered, How could anyone possibly drink so much orange juice?

Before I could recover from the shock of the super-jumbo orange juice, I saw a student cut up several thick layers of pancakes and pour syrup over them until they were completely drenched, soaked, and luxuriating in puddles of the sweet, sticky liquid. Lifting a large mouthful of pancake and syrup to his lips, he began to make his way quickly and methodically through the contents of his plate, first a bite of pancake, then a bite of the strips of grilled bacon on the side, then more pancake, until in a very short time everything was gone.

Nobody ate like this in Japan, and I assumed I never would either. Little did I know this was the beginning of my journey through the American way of serving and eating, or more precisely, the beginning of My Fat Years.

Though I loved practically everything about America, the food was at first an unpleasant jolt to my system. Japanese food and Japanese portions were what I grew up on, but Lewis University was in rural Illinois, and there were no Japanese restaurants or Japanese ingredients nearby.

Suddenly I was dropped into a culture and a daily life where the food was completely different and the portions seemed to me to be almost freakishly huge. Breakfast in the school cafeteria was piles of waffles soaked in oceans of syrup, flanked by boatloads of eggs and bacon. Lunch was giant cheeseburgers, fries, and soda, and dinner was mountains of meat and potatoes, heaps of pasta, and pizzas so big I could skate on them.

Nonetheless, I was thrilled to be transported to this completely foreign, brand-new environment. I loved everyone's classic American open, friendly, and happy attitude.

My English got better through "total immersion," and my gestures became less shy. My mannerisms became more casual. I started to chime into my girlfriends' conversations. I became so American I started to dream only in English. Even people who did not speak English in real life, like my parents, spoke in English in my dreams.

And soon I started to eat like my American friends too.

The result: within a few months of arriving in America, I had gained 25 pounds.

When I landed at O'Hare, I weighed not much more than

100 pounds (and stood five feet tall). Now I was pushing 125 pounds and bursting out of most of the clothes I had brought from Tokyo, especially my tight jeans.

I tried to work off the extra calories by running on a stretch of field behind the dorm. But it was in vain: I couldn't lose an ounce. Soon it was winter and the Chicago area seemed buried in snow for half the year. I stayed indoors most of the winter. I got very little exercise.

I was invited to visit local American families, and everything they served was delicious. But I was staggered by the size of the portions and by how much bread, meat, and potatoes was considered normal. It seemed that Americans were used to consuming at least twice as much food at every meal as we did in Japan.

Then came the dessert. To my astonishment, it consisted not of a single course, but several: apple pies, pecan pies, pumpkin pies, chocolate pies—often two or more different kinds—and cookies, too. From the freezers emerged gigantic buckets of ice cream: vanilla, chocolate, mint chocolate chip, and strawberry. Honestly, in Japan you'd never see so much ice cream in one place. What an incredibly wealthy country, I marveled; they eat tons of ice cream even in the freezing winter!

When I wasn't invited to people's homes, I learned to eat typical college fare. Soon my diet revolved around pizza, pies, cookies, and ice cream. I loved fully loaded Burger King Whoppers.

But I wasn't completely happy with what I was eating. I wrote a letter to my parents confessing my huge craving for what I missed most: lightly cooked and lightly seasoned Japanese home-style fresh vegetables, and boiled Napa cabbage.

Despite gaining 25 pounds and missing veggies, I was

thrilled to be going to school, making friends, and acquiring American habits. Weeks and months went by fast. I spent two years in the Midwest without ever going back to Japan. Finally, after many happy days in the midst of the cornfields of Illinois, I returned home.

My family came to meet me at the airport and I immediately began gushing about how much I loved America.

One of my aunts interrupted with a blunt question: "How could you be so happy there? Look at you—you got fat!" She was right.

Living in Tokyo again, I went through reverse culture shock. Tokyo is super-dense and crowded: streets are narrow, apartments are tiny, and commuter trains are packed (commuters are literally packed and squeezed into rush hour trains by uniformed men with white gloves). I had grown used to the wide-open spaces of the American Midwest.

I went back to live with my parents, since it's customary in Japan even now for single people to stay home until they get married. With my now fluent English, I found a job as an English-Japanese translator at Tokyo Disneyland.

Then, in a matter of a few weeks, something incredible happened.

Between the walking-intensive Tokyo lifestyle and my mother's home cooking, the extra 25 pounds began to miraculously melt away. I didn't do anything conscious to lose the weight; I simply went back to my mother's Tokyo kitchen and the Japanese urban way of life.

And suddenly one day I found I could easily fit into all my old clothes.

After a stint at Tokyo Disneyland, I went to work at Grey

Advertising in Tokyo, where I thought I might enjoy a profession that combines commerce and creativity. I did enjoy it, but I missed life in the United States. Before long, I begged my bosses to send me to New York, and they gave in.

Once ensconced in my new office at Grey Advertising's headquarters on Third Avenue, I worked on the Kraft General Foods and Procter & Gamble accounts.

My first apartment in Manhattan had a tiny kitchen with a big refrigerator, a big oven, a sink, and cupboards. There was no space to chop or prepare foods, and no ventilation for cooking fish. I asked a colleague at the office, "What's up with these Manhattan kitchens? They don't give you any space to prepare food. And what am I supposed to do with this refrigerator?"

She said, "Well, most of us in New York go out to eat, bring a doggie bag home, put it in the refrigerator, and heat it up in the oven the next day."

Wow, that makes sense, I thought. I like the efficiency!

So I became a happy Manhattan junior executive—slaving at work, writing memos, crunching numbers, partying with friends, getting no sleep, and having a great time.

When I went back to Tokyo to visit my family, my mother, in her typical fashion, asked, "Are you eating well?"

"Of course, Mom, I live in New York! Lots of fabulous restaurants and take-out places. Plus, I have a microwave oven!"

"What do you mean you have a microwave oven?" My mother despaired. "Does it mean that you do not have pots and pans? That you're only eating takeout? That you do not cook?"

When I turned around, my mom was shoving a frying pan in my suitcase, exclaiming, "Take this with you!"

I said, "Mom, I can buy a pan in America too!"

But the difference between what I was used to at home in Tokyo and in my New York life went beyond home-cooked versus takeout and microwaved meals. From childhood, Japanese are accustomed to eating portions that are a third smaller than or even half of American portions. And while Americans often eat until they feel completely satiated (or beyond), there is a Japanese mother's saying that recommends *"Hara hachi bunme"*—or "Eat until you are 80 percent full."

In Japan, food is meant to be eaten slowly, and every bite should be savored. But here's the beautiful part—after a good Japanese-style home-cooked meal, you shouldn't feel hungry at all!

Japanese learn these habits almost from birth, at home and school. In a typical Japanese elementary school, there are no buffet-style cafeterias or vending machines. Instead, kids eat communally in the classroom and take turns *serving one another,* wearing special serving hats and smocks. Each child is served the same amount of the same dish (you can ask for seconds).

In Japan, meals are served on plates, bowls, and dishes that are almost bite-size compared with their American counterparts. This greatly reduces portion sizes and enhances the food's aesthetic and spiritual appeal.

If you are invited to a Japanese home for dinner, you're in for quite a memorable event. In 1933, the great German architect Bruno Taut came to Japan and left us with a written account of a beautiful meal he had in a Japanese home. The experience, he wrote, was "highly aesthetic": "Various dishes were laid on the table, each in its own receptacle. Broth was in a lacquer bowl, and for fish there was a plate of irregular shape, decorated with a glaze of a very subdued color that blended well with that of the bowl." There was a plate for red and white slices of raw fish, plus a covered bowl of rice and a little wine cup. "My wife in particular was wonderstruck at the beauty of the repast spread out before us," he remembered. "It would appear that the appetite of the Japanese is aroused principally through appeal to his optic nerves."

The basic foundations of Japanese home-cooked food presentation are:

- never completely fill up the plates
- never serve a big portion of any item
- each item is served in its own dish
- less is always more
- each item is arranged to showcase its natural beauty
- food should be garnished and dressed—lightly
- fresh is best

The importance of "empty" space in the presentation of Japanese cuisine can scarcely be exaggerated. Receptacles are never filled to the brim, but are left with a certain margin of emptiness—emptiness of an aesthetic significance comparable to that in Zen ink painting.

—Chef Masaru Yamamoto

Chilled Tofu with Bonito Flakes and Chopped Scallions

SERVES 4

Silken tofu is the rich, creamy star of this cool summer dish. Simple yet completely delightful, this is a perfect illustration of Japanese-style portion control, a food painting so beautiful and so delicately tasty that it demands to be savored with both eyes and mouth.

> One 8-ounce block of silken tofu, mildly chilled
> 2 teaspoons freshly toasted and ground white sesame seeds (page 111)
> 1 teaspoon minced fresh mitsuba (page 151) or Italian parsley
> 1 shiso leaf, cut into very thin ribbons
> Reduced-sodium soy sauce, to use at the table
> ¼ cup small bonito flakes
> 2 teaspoons minced scallion, roots and top cut off

1. Gently rinse the chilled tofu under cold water and drain well.
2. Arrange the garnishes. Ground sesame seeds can be placed in a small shallow bowl with a tiny spoon for serving. Put the minced mitsuba and slivered shiso leaf on a small plate. Bring these garnishes to the table, along with a bottle of reduced-sodium soy sauce.
3. Prepare the tofu by carefully cutting the block into four equal

pieces, making sure to keep the pieces intact—and beautiful. Place each block on a small plate and top with a portion of the bonito flakes and minced scallion. Let diners further season their tofu as desired with the herbs, ground sesame seeds, and some soy.

Tokyo Kitchen Tip

Serve the tofu mildly cold, not too chilled, so that you can taste and enjoy its flavor and texture.

SECRET 3
Japanese cooking is super-light and ultra-gentle.

Japanese wives and mothers cook food very lightly.

Traditionally, Japanese women didn't have ovens. Even now, while Westernized dishes like spaghetti and meatballs and salads are prepared, there is very little roasting or baking of large dishes at home, since Japanese kitchens are cramped, and the ovens are small. (My mother's Tokyo kitchen is really a one-woman kitchen—if she's in it, there's barely room for me.)

Instead of roasting or baking, Japanese women usually gently steam, pan-grill, sauté, simmer, or stir-fry quickly over medium or medium-high heat. These methods have the advantage of saving more of the food's nutrients.

Japanese women use subtle flavorings. Instead of smothering dishes in heavy cream or butter-based sauces, or seasoning them with overpowering spices, Japanese home chefs have a light, understated approach.

The whole idea of Japanese home cooking is to highlight the natural beauty and colors and let the essence of the food shine through.

The best cooking is the least cooking.

—Chizuko Moriyama

Here's another huge difference: instead of using dollops of animal fat, butter, or heavy oils, Japanese women cook with small, healthy doses of canola oil, or with dashi. A fish-and-sea-vegetable stock that is the secret ingredient of every Japanese home chef, dashi is a clear amber liquid resulting from the beautiful marriage between shaved bonito fish flakes and dried kombu, or kelp (see Bonito Flakes on page 93 and Sea Vegetables on page 106). It is one of the building blocks of Japanese home cooking, providing a delicate, mouthwatering alternative to stocks made from beef or chicken.

Japanese home cooks use dashi as a base in which to simmer food, as well as for soups, sauces, and dressings. Master chef Shizuo Tsuji, author of *Japanese Cooking: A Simple Art,* wrote, "Dashi provides Japanese cuisine with its characteristic flavor, and it can be said without exaggeration that the success or failure (or mediocrity) of a dish is ultimately determined by the flavor and quality of the dashi that seasons it."

The miracle of dashi lies in its ability to add a savory succulence to simmered dishes while liberating the essential flavors of each ingredient. To me, a potato tastes more like a potato when it's been simmered in dashi. The same holds true for eggplant, string beans, and almost any kind of fish.

In a *New York Times* article, food writer Mark Bittman described dashi as providing "a beguiling fragrance that is an odd combination of earth, sea, and smoke." If you've ever eaten an exquisite hot Japanese meal in a restaurant, chances are that dashi played a key behind-the-scenes role.

There are two versions of dashi. "First dashi" is the premium stock that results from using the kombu and fish flakes for the first time. Because it's very refined, this is the dashi used for clear soups and delicate simmered dishes.

"Second dashi" is the stock that results from simmering the "used" kombu and fish flakes in the same volume of water. Although not as delicate as first dashi, it's perfect for everyday miso soups and simmered dishes containing bold-tasting ingredients.

———

First Dashi

MAKES 4 CUPS

One 4-x-4-inch sheet kombu
4½ cups cold water
4 cups large bonito flakes (for a lighter taste you can
   use as little as 2 cups)

1. Place the sheet of kombu in a medium saucepan. Do not wash or wipe off the whitish powder on the seaweed's surface; it abounds with natural minerals and flavor. Add the cold water to the saucepan and bring the mixture almost to a boil. Immediately remove the kombu (saving it for making second dashi) to avoid the liquid's becoming bitter.

2. Add the bonito flakes and heat the liquid on high. When the

stock returns to a boil, immediately turn off the heat and let the flakes rest in the liquid for 2 minutes. Pour the stock through a fine-mesh sieve lined with cheesecloth. Avoid pressing on the flakes, to prevent the stock's becoming cloudy and bitter. (Save the bonito flakes for second dashi.)

3. Store the dashi in the refrigerator for up to 2 days (it spoils quickly).

Second Dashi

MAKES 4 CUPS

Combine the "used" kombu and bonito flakes from making the first dashi in a medium saucepan. Add 4½ cups of cold water and bring the mixture to a boil. Reduce the heat to low and simmer for 10 minutes. Pour the stock through a fine-mesh sieve lined with cheesecloth, discarding the solids this time. Store the dashi in the refrigerator for up to 2 days.

As a substitute for either first or second dashi, you can try instant dashi, which comes in granule, pouch, or liquid form. Look for an MSG-free version in Asian grocery stores or online. It's not quite as tasty as fresh homemade dashi, but it can save you time.

SECRET 4
The Japanese eat rice instead of bread with every meal.

A sandwich for lunch has become popular in Japan, as well as a piece of toast with breakfast. Today there are more than five thousand bakeries around Japan, offering goodies like Italian panini, French baguettes, and American bagels along with "Japanized" offerings like melon-pan sweetbread.

But overall, bread consumption in Japan is much lower than in the West, and rice is still the mainstay of the diet. Japanese people eat a medium portion of rice with almost every home-cooked meal. By having rice with most meals, the Japanese are able to avoid the belly-busting muffins, rolls, and white bread that are almost ubiquitous in America and are often eaten several times a day.

Japanese-Style Rice

MAKES 3 CUPS

Stove-Top Method

2 cups short-grain white rice, or haiga-mai, or brown
   rice
2 ½ cups cold water for white rice or haiga-mai; 3 cups
   for brown rice

1. Wash the rice (unless you are using haiga-mai) by putting the grains in a medium bowl and adding cold water to cover. Swish the grains with your hand to remove the starch and then drain off the cloudy water by tilting the bowl and holding the rice in the bowl with a cupped palm. Repeat this process two or three more times, or until the water when agitated around the rice is almost clear.

Drain the rice in a fine-mesh sieve. (Some brands of rice do not require washing; please read directions on the package.)

2. To cook the rice, transfer the washed grains to a medium saucepan. Add the 2½ cups of cold water (3 cups for brown rice) and let the rice sit in the water 20 minutes to plump. Cover the saucepan and bring the rice to a boil. Reduce the heat to low and gently simmer the rice for 15 minutes (longer for brown rice) or until all liquid is evaporated. Turn off the heat and let the rice sit, covered, for 10 minutes. When ready to serve, fluff the rice grains by gently turning them over with a wet wooden paddle or spatula.

Electric Rice Cooker Method (Makes 3 cups)

2 cups short-grain Japanese rice
Cold water

1. Wash the rice according to the instructions indicated above for the Stove-Top Method.
2. To cook the rice, transfer the washed grains to the cooking bowl of an electric rice cooker. Add enough cold water to the bowl, according to the machine's instructions, for 2 cups of dry rice. Let the rice sit in the water 20 minutes to plump. Plug in the rice cooker and push the On or Start button. When the rice has finished cooking, let it rest undisturbed for 10 minutes (do not open the lid). When ready to serve, fluff the rice grains by gently turning them over with a wet wooden paddle or spatula.

SECRET 5

Japanese women are the princesses of power breakfast.

Japanese women don't eat pancakes for breakfast.

They don't eat piles of eggs and bacon.

They don't eat bagels and cream cheese, blueberry muffins, or sugary cereals.

Poor things, you may think. How deprived—and how sad they must feel!

But wait a minute—take a look at their waistlines—they are the low-obesity champions of the industrialized world!

And one of the reasons is that Japanese women are the princesses of power breakfast.

Every morning across Japan, millions of wives and mothers are whipping up a Japanese home-cooked breakfast for themselves and their families. A typical breakfast in Japan consists of green tea, a bowl of steamed rice, miso soup with tofu and scallions, small sheets of nori seaweed, and perhaps a small omelette or piece of grilled salmon.

One Japanese mother, Sawako Cline, explains: "In Japan, breakfast is the most important and often biggest meal of the day. I will get up earlier and spend thirty minutes making it for my kids. Sometimes we will have fish or rice and miso soup, sometimes ham and eggs with vegetables and always fruit."

Every morning in New York, I have a breakfast of low-sodium miso soup, usually containing one egg, scallions, tofu, a spoonful of brown rice, and assorted little chopped vegetables or tomatoes left over from the night before.

Give it a try and see how fantastic you feel—all the way through to lunch!

Japanese Country Power Breakfast

SERVES 4

I adapted this hearty miso soup recipe from my grandmother Tsune Moriyama, who made it for breakfast every time my family visited my father's ancestral home in the countryside. My favorite part was always the whole egg. Over the years, my husband, Billy, and I have added more vegetables to the base, along with tofu and rice to make it the "power breakfast" we eat nearly every morning in New York. A bowl of this soup in the morning fuels me right through the day. It's satisfying but not heavy.

½ cup hot cooked rice (page 54)

4 large eggs

½ of a 3-x-5-inch block atsu-age tofu (thick-fried tofu)

12 grape tomatoes, or 8 cherry tomatoes

2 scallions, roots and top cut off, with white and green parts thinly sliced and kept separate from each other

1 cup mixed cooked vegetables (such as string beans, carrots, and corn)

4 cups dashi (page 52)

2½ tablespoons red or white miso (or use a combination of both)

1. Place the eggs in a small saucepan with water to cover. Bring to a boil and cook for 7 minutes. Remove the eggs with a

slotted spoon and put them on a plate so they can cool.
When cool enough to handle, peel and quarter each egg.

2. Bring water to a boil in a small saucepan. Add the atsu-age tofu
   and gently boil over medium heat, turning occasionally, for 1
   minute; drain (this will remove excess oil). Cut the tofu into
   small squares.

3. Lay out 4 small soup bowls. In each one arrange a portion of
   egg wedges, fried tofu squares, the white part of the sliced scallions, tomatoes, cooked vegetables, and cooked rice.

4. Place the dashi in a large saucepan and bring to a boil. Whisk
   in the miso and turn off the heat. Ladle the hot miso broth over
   the ingredients in the bowls. Garnish each serving with the
   reserved green part of the scallions.

SECRET 6
Japanese women are crazy for dessert . . . in a special way.

Japanese women are crazy for chocolate.

They love their pastries, ice cream, cookies, rice crackers,
and red-bean cakes.

The difference is that they eat desserts and snacks less often
and in (you guessed it) smaller portions. A typical piece of
cake is one third the size of an American slice.

Gourmet-quality chocolate can be found everywhere in
Japan, and some of the bakeries in Tokyo are on a par with the
finest bakeries in Paris. There are donut shops in all Japanese
cities. But the Japanese people have never fallen into the habit of
eating big desserts, and they're happy to enjoy just 25 percent of the
quantity of confectionary products per capita that Americans eat.

Let me tell you a story: When my sister, Miki, was three or

four, she went through a phase where she barely ate meals and got very skinny. She would push the food around on her plate, take a few small bites, and say that she was done.

My mother worried that Miki was not getting enough nutrition. She knew that some mothers in our neighborhood gave kids sweets, and she thought that if she could make sure that Miki didn't eat any between-meal snacks, Miki would be more likely to eat what she was served at home. So my mother pinned a small sign on my little sister that read:

Please do not feed me any sweets or food.

I think Miki was too young to read and didn't understand what the sign meant.

Years later, I saw the great Japanese movie about food, *Tampopo,* in which there was a scene that showed a small Japanese boy wandering around a playground with a hand lettered wooden sign hanging from his neck. On the sign was a drawing of a carrot and the warning:

Do not feed me sweets. I eat only natural food.

Once again, my mother was ahead of her time!

SECRET 7
Japanese women have a different relationship with food.

There may be another reason that Japanese women are both the world's longevity champions and the industrial world's low-obesity champions: *a healthier relationship with food.*

While there is a growing problem of eating disorders among younger Japanese women, it seems that overall, Japanese may still eat more healthfully than people in the West.

In a 2003 report on eating habits, researchers at Brigham Young University found that Americans have a "less healthy relationship with food" than the Japanese. "Ironically, the American premium on thinness and the focus on dietary restriction and deprivation are possibly the important contributors to the growing rates of obesity, emotional eating, eating disorders and poor body image in the United States," reported Associate Professor of Health Science Steve Hawks, the lead researcher for the study.

"Americans primarily associate food with health objectives such as being thin and least with the simple pleasure of a satisfying meal," said Hawks. "The Japanese, on the other hand, have managed to maintain a more healthy relationship with food in terms of diversity of diet and less of a focus on the restriction and deprivation that go along with trying to be thin."

The study found that Japanese women do place a high value on thinness, but they don't seem to deny themselves favorite foods to the same extent as American women. "This heavy degree of restrictive dieting in America may actually

A good, functional and healthy body is the ultimate fashion statement.

—Kiyokazu Washida,
fashion critic

lead to increased obesity," Hawks reported. "The body reacts to dieting by storing more fat than normal and by significantly decreasing the number of calories burned during normal activities."

THE JAPANESE MINI OBESITY CRISIS

You may be thinking, Wait a minute. It's easy for Japanese to be slim. They can't get fat—it's in their genes!

I don't think this explains why so few Japanese are obese, for three reasons.

Reason #1: myself. I am 100 percent ethnically Japanese, and whenever I stop eating Japanese-style food and portions and start eating the wrong foods and big portions, I start packing on pounds with frightening speed. In other words, I get *fat*.

Reason #2: science. Research indicates that when Japanese leave Japan and start eating typical Western food and portions, their health suffers. According to Professor Kerin O'Dea, director of the Menzies School of Health Research in Australia, "health studies of migrant populations (Hawaii and the U.S.) indicate that Japanese are at least as susceptible to cardiovascular diseases and diet-related cancers when they live a more Westernised lifestyle—and diet has been the major factor implicated in such studies."

Experts also believe that diet has a direct impact upon longevity. A leading British authority on aging, Professor Tom Kirkwood of the University of Newcastle, considers that some three quarters of the human aging process is influenced by nongenetic factors that we can control, such as nutrition and lifestyle. He notes that "Japanese who change to a 'Western' diet age faster and experience the disease profile typical of Western societies."

Reason #3 is, in my opinion, the most persuasive reason— right now, inside Japan itself, as Japanese eat more and more Western-style food, the nation is starting to suffer a mini obesity crisis.

"The Japanese are getting fatter, just as we are," says Professor Marion Nestle, an obesity and nutrition expert at New York University, "although they are still a few years behind." As some Japanese become more sedentary and eat more high-calorie junk food, Professor Nestle says, "they too are gaining weight—especially kids." This certainly looks like a dangerous trend, which may blossom into a major crisis in Japan if it isn't stopped.

To me, the commonsense conclusion is pretty obvious: when Japanese people abandon the traditional Japanese diet and eat a typical Western-style, less healthy diet, they get fat, just like everybody else. It looks like genes are little protection against a fat-promoting diet and lifestyle.

AN EXTRA JAPANESE SECRET
Japanese exercise throughout the day—naturally.

Food isn't the only reason that Japanese are living so long and so healthy. Another factor is the automatic workout they get in their everyday lives. "The Japanese are in good health and in excellent shape," announced *Time* magazine in a 2004 cover story, "How to Live to Be 100." The reason is that "they are an active people who incorporate plenty of incidental exercise into their days."

Japanese seniors are especially active. Makoto Suzuki, a professor at Okinawa International University, said, "As opposed to America, seniors in Japan do not have to purposely go out and seek exercise—everyday life makes them more slim and healthy." Along with nutritious eating habits, he noted, "It's a winning combination."

Take my family, for instance. Not only does my mother, Chizuko, crisscross the streets of Tokyo on foot all day, often dashing up and down flights of stairs, but on weekends she goes hiking in the mountains with her buddies. Last summer, my parents took Billy and me on a hike up Mt. Takao, a 1,969-foot hill in a national park west of Tokyo. When we got to the summit after a ninety-minute climb, my mother announced matter-of-factly, "I'm not tired at all!"

Like tens of millions of Japanese, my father, Shigeo, who is in his early seventies, gets around the neighborhood on a basic old-fashioned bicycle. It's not exactly a Lance Armstrong high-tech bike: in fact it's a one-speed. He regularly bikes over to my sister's house twenty blocks away to babysit his grandchildren.

In turn, my sister, Miki, rides her bicycle all around town, sometimes with groceries in the front basket and one of my nieces, four-year-old Kasumi or two-year-old Ayaka, riding in the child seat behind her. She often picks up my six-year-old nephew, Kazuma, at school the same way—on the bike. Miki's husband, Shiko, is even more active, because he's in an exercise-intense line of work: he's a leading instructor of classical Japanese dance and conducts dance classes around the country.

On narrow streets and sidewalks all over Tokyo, you'll see businessmen making their rounds on bicycles, and women on bikes running errands and going grocery shopping. And what happens in Tokyo holds true throughout the nation.

Lined up outside every train station in Japan, you'll notice rows upon rows of parked bicycles that belong to commuters. One of them belongs to my uncle Kazuo, who is in his early seventies and commutes to Tokyo from a suburb. Rain or shine, every weekday you'll see him leaving home and pedaling over to the station to park his bike and board the train, a dapper figure in his suit and tie.

"What happens when it rains?" I asked him.

He gave me a broad grin: "Why, then I just hold the umbrella in one hand, and the bike with the other!" His wife, Yoshiko, swims every day and is a scuba-diving buff.

The simple act of taking the subway in Tokyo is itself a workout. The stations are sprawling, mazelike affairs, requiring lots of stair climbing and walking between the different subway lines to transfer.

In addition to "incidental" everyday exercise, lots of Japanese are getting out there and deliberately working up a sweat.

Every morning in Tokyo at the crack of dawn, you'll see a lean hundred-year-old man named Keizo Miura pounding the pavement for a power walk, before a breakfast of eggs and seaweed. At age ninety-nine he skied down Mont Blanc in the Italian Alps.

In 2003 his son, seventy-two-year-old Yuichiro Miura, became the oldest man ever to climb Mount Everest—a year after his fellow Japanese Tamae Watanabe became, at sixty-three, the oldest woman to scale the mountain.

"Older Japanese are remarkably healthy, doing things at

their age that most youngsters couldn't do," the younger Mr. Miura told a visiting reporter doing a story on Japanese longevity. "People over sixty-five here are climbing mountains, going to China to plant trees, traveling abroad to teach Japanese. It's about diet, it's about exercise, it's about making the most out of a long life."

In the summer of 2005, a seventy-one-year-old Japanese man named Minoru Saito stunned the sailing world when he became the oldest man to circumnavigate the planet solo, without stopping at a single port.

While these people are at the extremes of fitness, keeping active and strong is part of the Japanese lifestyle, and the Japanese love recreational sports. Popular sports around the country include golf, soccer, baseball, tennis, snowboarding, and skiing, as well as martial arts like karate, judo, and kendo. The fitness ethos is part of the workplace too: many Japanese factories and companies encourage their employees to begin their days with exercise, such as a twenty-minute rooftop workout.

This is not to say there aren't millions of stressed-out, nonexercising people in Japan who are smoking and drinking their way to early graves. However, Dr. Lawrence Kushi, associate research director for the Kaiser Permanente health care plan in California, who has studied diet and exercise patterns of Japanese and Westerners, notes that Japanese people "are much more active in their daily lives than most Europeans, Australians, and definitely people in the United States. They are much more likely to walk substantial distances, bicycle, or climb stairs in their daily activities, and much less likely to drive."

The health benefits of walking are highly praised by experts—and backed up by solid research. "Exercise can cut the risk of developing heart disease by half as well as lowering blood pressure, reducing stress and minimizing the risk of strokes," Professor Charles George, medical director for the British Heart Foundation, told a journalist for *The Express*. "Since walking is one of the easiest, most convenient and inexpensive forms of exercise, it's an excellent choice for many people."

One hot walking trend is "10,000 steps." This idea was first popularized forty years ago by a Japanese researcher named Yoshiro Hatano as a way of promoting the first cheap, reliable pedometer. Today, the goal of walking 10,000 steps a day (about five miles) is supported by groups like the Centers for Disease Control and Prevention and the American College of Sports Medicine.

"We do have good cross-sectional studies showing that people who walk 10,000 steps per day are leaner and have lower blood pressure than those who walk less," declared Professor David Bassett of the University of Tennessee on NPR's *Morning Edition* on May 16, 2005. The executive director of the President's Council on Physical Fitness, Melissa Johnson, agreed: "Ten thousand steps is a phenomenal goal for people to shoot for."

In New York City, concrete streets are my exercise machine. I try to walk everywhere around town. I walk several miles a day to and from the office, and Billy and I often take a long walk to the Union Square farmers market and jog around the Central Park Reservoir on weekends.

Take a tip from millions of Japanese natural health nuts—lace up your sneakers and hit the walking trail!

CHAPTER 4

How to Start Your Tokyo Kitchen
or, Yes, You Can Do This at Home!

Mommy, I want Japanese for dinner!

—A seven-year-old American boy in New York's
Central Park, January 5, 2005

How EASY *IS* IT to start your own Tokyo kitchen?

Guess what—you probably already have one!

Chances are, right now in your kitchen, you've got much of what you need to start making Japanese home-cooked food.

There isn't a huge amount of difference between a well-stocked American kitchen and a Tokyo kitchen. Many of the tools are the same or almost identical. You probably have most of the equipment in your kitchen already, and the new ingredients you'll need are available at the supermarket, or are just a few clicks away.

To see how close your kitchen is to a Tokyo kitchen, consider what happened to my mother when she visited New York.

In 2002 my mother and her sister, my aunt Yoshiko, came from Tokyo to spend a few weeks in New York to do some sightseeing and shopping. My mother wanted to try living a New York lifestyle rather than staying in a hotel. So Billy and I rented them a furnished apartment in our neighborhood in midtown New York. The apartment had a typical wide-open American kitchen, without any uniquely Japanese-style utensils or equipment.

Walking into the apartment, my mother was overjoyed to see how big the kitchen was compared with her miniature Tokyo workspace. Within minutes of arriving and checking out the equipment in the kitchen, she and my aunt (neither of whom speaks English) were out on their own, bargaining with the local fruit and vegetable stand proprietor on Second Avenue, and patrolling the aisles of a nearby chain supermarket in search of rice, eggs, and soy sauce. They didn't go to a special Japanese market—although they could have, because we have a number of them not far away—and they did not buy any utensils to add to the standard items supplied by the rental apartment.

The next day, my mother whipped up a fantastic meal starring one of her home-cooked original dishes, which she calls Iri Iri Pan Pan, otherwise known as Super-Scrambled Eggs and Beef. It's a yin-yang presentation of finely scrambled eggs next to chopped beef gently sautéed in soy sauce. Billy nearly passed out, it tasted so good.

My mother and Aunt Yoshiko wound up cooking almost

every day they were in New York, finding most of what they needed right in their neighborhood, and working in a Western kitchen that is probably similar to your own.

The moral of this story is: You don't have to live in Tokyo to do this at home!

———

Iri Iri Pan Pan
a.k.a. Mom's Super-Scrambled Eggs and Ground Beef

SERVES 4

My mother often comes up with her own nicknames for things. For example, she calls a microwave oven "chin" for the sound it makes at the end of the cooking process, and she uses it as a verb, as in "please chin the rice for 30 seconds," and as a noun, as in "you can put it in the chin." This scrambled-eggs-and-beef dish is familiar to anyone in Japan, except for its name, "Iri Iri Pan Pan," which is another of my mother's inventions. "Iri Iri," according to her, describes the constant action of scrambling necessary to making this dish a success, and "Pan Pan" is the sound the saucepan makes as it is moved around during the scrambling.

The bright yellow eggs in this dish contrast beautifully with the rich brown beef and the vivid green pea pod strips, and the flavor combinations, simple as they are, are breathtaking.

Super-Scrambled Eggs

1 tablespoon canola oil or rice bran oil
6 large eggs
2 tablespoon granulated sugar
Pinch of salt

Super-Scrambled Ground Beef

1 tablespoon canola oil or rice bran oil
1 pound finely ground extra lean ground beef (ask your
    butcher to grind 2 to 3 extra times, or give it those
    extra grinds at home in your food processor)
2 tablespoon sake
1 tablespoon sugar
1 tablespoon reduced-sodium soy sauce
Pinch of salt

8 snow pea pods, stems trimmed
4 cups of cooked brown or white rice (page 54)

1. Heat 1 tablespoon canola oil or rice bran oil in a small
   saucepan. Add the eggs and sugar to the saucepan, bring heat
   to medium, and scramble the eggs with a wooden cooking
   fork, or a whisk, for 2 minutes. When the eggs start to harden,
   add the pinch of salt. Continue to scramble for 2 more minutes, or until the eggs are just cooked and in very small pieces.
   Remove the eggs from the pan and set aside.
2. Heat 1 tablespoon canola oil or rice bran oil in a small
   saucepan. Add the ground beef, sake, sugar, soy sauce, and salt
   to the saucepan, and bring heat to medium. Sauté the beef,
   stirring constantly with a wooden cooking fork to keep the beef

in constant motion so that it never clumps, for 6 minutes or until cooked through. Remove from pan and set aside.

3. Bring a small saucepan of water to a boil. Add the snow peas and cook over medium-high heat for 1 minute, or until they are crisp-tender. Drain and refresh under cold water. Cut the pods lengthwise into julienne strips.

4. Lay out 4 medium bowls. Scoop 1 cup cooked rice into each bowl with a wet spatula, then gently smooth out the surface so that the bed of rice is relatively flat (not mounded, but not packed tight either). Spoon one quarter of the super-scrambled eggs over the left half of the rice in each bowl, one quarter of the beef mixture over the right half, and spread eggs and beef evenly over their respective sides. Divide the snow pea strips into 4 equal portions and place them in the middle of each bowl, where the eggs and beef meet.

Tokyo Kitchen Tips

The smaller the pieces of eggs and beef, the more elegant the texture and appearance of this dish.

Using small saucepans makes it easier to scramble without over-cooking.

To maximize the beauty of this dish, keep scrambling even if your arm wants to quit.

———

It is easy to start your own Tokyo kitchen. You already have 90 percent of the things you need.

The remaining 10 percent consists of two basic pieces of equipment, some Japanese-style dishes, and a short shopping list of basic ingredients. And if you prefer, you can even skimp on the equipment and tableware.

Of course, as with anything else in life, like carpentry or gardening, you could go totally crazy and acquire a wide range of obscure and highly authentic special tools and utensils to start Japanese-style home cooking. But you wouldn't need most of them. As my friend David, who studied French cooking in Paris, once said, "I do not believe in having extra cooking utensils. If a teaspoon does the job, I don't need a measuring spoon."

For basic Japanese home cooking, many Western cooking utensils and ingredients will do just fine, as long as they are high-quality. The question is not whether your knife or frying pan is American or Japanese. What matters is whether your knife is sharp and cuts well, and your frying pan and skillet distribute heat evenly and fast. Chopping vegetables with a dull knife is no fun, and sautéing food at heat that is not high enough means that the foods lose their color. With high heat, vegetables and other foods stay bright and beautiful.

If you have a food processor, so much the better. That's great for mincing, shredding, and grating, which are often required for Japanese home cooking.

With a few key exceptions, my mother's Tokyo kitchen looks a lot like a miniature Western-style kitchen. And believe it or not, you can probably find many of the items used in a Tokyo kitchen—in your own kitchen.

THE TOKYO KITCHEN YOU ALREADY HAVE

Equipment
> Pots in various sizes: aluminum, cast iron, copper, enamel,
> earthenware, stainless steel
> Frying pans in various sizes

Steamer

Strainer

Vegetable cutter, grater and/or zester

Universal knife

Vegetable knife

Cutting board

Wood or rubber spatula

Ladle

Whisk

Tongs

Measuring spoon and cup

Kitchen carver

Flat wooden spoon

Mixing bowls

Sieve

Food processor

Tableware

Serving plates, bowls, and platters

Place settings of bowls and plates

Condiment, snack, and dipping dishes

Flatware

Teapot, cups, and mugs

Ingredients and Seasonings

Sugar

Salt

Pepper

Gingerroot

To add to this basic foundation, you need a few more essentials to get started. The great news is you can get many of the utensils and tableware items at stores like Target, Bed Bath & Beyond, and Crate & Barrel, Pottery Barn, and Wal-Mart, or from QVC, eBay, or Amazon.

The foods you can find at stores like Whole Foods, Wild Oats, Safeway, Kroger, Food Emporium, Albertsons, and— if you're lucky enough to live near one—at your local Japanese or Asian market. Some of them you can also get online.

SHOPPING CHECKLIST TO COMPLETE YOUR TOKYO KITCHEN

New Equipment (Optional)
Rice cooker
Wok

New Tableware (Optional)
Japanese teaware: teapot, teacups, and saucers
Japanese- or Asian-style tableware
    One 2- to 3-inch ceramic or earthenware soy sauce cruet
    One slightly larger sauce-serving ceramic or earthenware pitcher
      for tempura and other sauces
    Several serving plates, bowls, and platters

    Basic place setting for each person
     • Rice bowl
     • Soup bowl
     • Two or three 3- to 5-inch-diameter dishes

- Two or three 3- to 5-inch-diameter, 1- to 3-inch deep bowls
- Two square or rectangular plates
- Three 2- to 3-inch-diameter condiment plates
- Hot noodle bowl
- Cold noodle tray with bamboo strainer
- Dipping sauce cup
- Chopsticks and chopstick rest

New Basic Ingredients and Seasonings (Essential)

Bonito (fish) flakes (katsuobushi, hana-katsuo, or kezuri-bushi)

Daikon (Japanese giant white radish)

Japanese-style short-grain rice

Japanese teas

Mirin (cooking wine)

Miso (fermented soybean paste)

Noodles: soba (buckwheat noodles) and udon (thick white flour noodles)

Oils: canola oil, rice bran oil, sesame oil

Rice vinegar

Rice wine (sake)

Sea vegetables: hijiki; kombu, konbu, or kobu (Japanese kelp); nori (laver)

Sesame seeds (goma)

Shiso

Soy sauce (shoyu)

Tofu

Wasabi

STARTER UTENSILS FOR YOUR TOKYO KITCHEN

Miracle Product 1: The Amazing Rice Cooker

How do Japanese women stay so healthy and slim?

One big reason is that they are world-champion rice eaters, sometimes eating a bowl of rice four times a day, for breakfast, lunch, dinner, and even as a snack. In Japan, rice often takes the place that bread, donuts, or even less healthy belly-fillers occupy in Western diets.

And how do so many Japanese women cook fluffy, perfect rice every day for themselves and their family? Like my mother, they use a magical invention called an automatic electric rice cooker.

Years ago, one of my American friends asked how I managed to make such delicious rice every single time. "It's simple," I told her. "I use an electric rice cooker. It's like a coffee machine. All you have to do is to put rice and water in it, and plug it in."

The automatic rice cooker was launched in 1955 in Japan, revolutionizing housewives' daily routines. Before that, people cooked rice in a heavy pot over a stove. Now you'll find a rice cooker in almost all Japanese home kitchens. It's one of my mother's most well-used kitchen tools. If you and your family plan to enjoy rice as a regular part of your diet (and I hope you do), it makes sense to invest in a rice cooker.

Today, in the West, electric rice cookers are becoming so popular that they show up on bridal registries. Thanks to the Internet, you can select a rice cooker from a wide range of brands, prices, and functions. A Google search for "rice cooker" yields 853,000 results, and its Froogle e-commerce section shows over 3,000 items that you can sort by price or store.

Specialty stores like Williams-Sonoma and Bed Bath & Beyond, department stores like Macy's, and mass merchandisers like Target carry many varieties. Most cost between $100 and $200.

A rice cooker saves you time, and it's failure-proof, consistently making rice that is moist yet fluffy with just a hint of stickiness but no gumminess. Most rice cookers come with a "warmer" function, so rice stays warm in the cooker throughout the day or even into the next day, allowing you to make enough rice for dinner and the following day's breakfast and lunch box. Most rice cookers also come with a nonstick pan, which is easy to clean.

Easy Rice Cooker Alternative: Cook rice in a pot on top of your stove.

If you're not quite ready to invest in a rice cooker, you can make rice simply by cooking it on top of the stove and following the instructions on the package. Most instructions call for bringing the rice to a boil, then reducing to a very low simmer and cooking until the water evaporates. Although it can sometimes be tricky to get the rice to come out exactly the way you like it—neither overcooked so that it's gummy and stuck together, nor undercooked and crunchy—so long as you're prepared to do a bit of experimenting and to have a possible mishap or two before you arrive at the proper technique, you'll soon nail down your own winning formula for delicious rice.

Miracle Product 2: The Trusty Wok

Since so much of Japanese home-style cooking involves quick, high-heat stir-frying, a wok—a cookware tool with an ancient

A HOT AND FLUFFY RICE TIP FROM TOKYO
Homemade Microwaveable Frozen Rice

Whether you use a rice cooker or a pot, a great time-saving trick is to make extra portions of rice while you're cooking your rice for dinner. Place the leftovers in a microwave-safe container while the rice is still fluffy and hot, and stick it in the freezer.

When you're ready for your next meal, microwave the container on medium power for 1 to 2 minutes (microwave powers differ, so please adjust accordingly) and serve. It's a great way to be able to enjoy rice when you don't have time to cook it.

Chinese lineage—is an indispensable, multipurpose piece of equipment.

Woks are about 10 to 14 inches in diameter, 3 to 4 inches deep, and usually round-bottomed. They're made of carbon steel or cast iron.

Besides stir-frying, you can sauté, boil, deep-fry, or steam in a wok. If you don't have Asian cookware yet, a wok should be one of the first things you buy to start enjoying the benefits of Japanese home-style cooking.

My mother has four woks. She uses them to sauté vegetables very quickly at high heat, so they don't lose either their nutrients or their beautiful bright colors: carrots stay orange, spinach deep green, and eggplant shiny purple. My mother also makes all kinds of other dishes in her wok, like Snap Peas, Daikon, and Egg Soup (page 95), fried rice (*cha-han*), and Shrimp and Vegetable Tempura (page 143).

The temperature in a wok can get much higher than in a flat frying pan. The hottest portion can be as high as 752°F, versus 536°F in a frying pan, according to an estimate by the Japanese Broadcasting Corporation. The curved bottom and wide surface area of the wok help distribute heat evenly all the way around and also makes it easy to flip the ingredients.

I use my wok to simmer ingredients and stir-fry vegetables. I also use it to steam vegetables by boiling water in it and stacking bamboo steamers over the water.

These days, you can pick up a great wok almost anywhere. Just like electric rice cookers, you can find many selections on the Internet, or at kitchen equipment specialty stores, department stores, and mass merchandisers. Authentic woks have a rounded bottom, but you can also find models with a flat bottom; these sit on flat-surfaced burners without tilting and are recommended for use on electric stoves.

Easy Wok Alternative: Use what you already have.

Until you get your own trusty wok, you can use a frying pan made of Calphalon, cast iron, or stainless-steel-clad aluminum or copper (all good sturdy heat conductors that can withstand high heat) for sautéing and stir-frying, a saucepan for simmering and boiling, and a deep, wide-rimmed skillet for deep-frying.

STARTER TABLEWARE FOR YOUR TOKYO KITCHEN

Since aesthetics are an integral part of Japanese home cooking, you may choose to buy some Japanese tableware to enhance your family's dining experiences.

Japanese Teaware: A Beautiful Accessory for Introducing Green Tea into Your Lifestyle

I hope that you'll consider adding healthy, delicious green tea to your lifestyle, and when you do, it's a great idea to get your own Japanese tea set.

By the way, I'm not talking about a Japanese tea *ceremony*. That's an elaborate, highly ritualized, and near spiritual celebration of tea that is beautiful to behold and partake in, but it's not what most Japanese people do every day in their homes.

Japanese men and women drink green tea all the time: with meals, between meals, as a morning perk-up and as an evening relaxer. (See page 98 for the varieties of Japanese green tea.) At restaurants in Japan, hot green tea is free, like tap water. Though green tea is the most common, the Japanese also drink black tea and, in summer, many drink cold barley tea (*mugicha*).

On a typical Japanese dining table, you'll see a tea set along with an airtight canister of loose green tea leaves and a pot filled with boiling water.

In America, people tend to have their own special personal coffee cups, which they use every time they have coffee. It's the same thing in Japan with teacups.

In the United States, a Japanese tea set for everyday use consists of a ceramic or cast-iron teapot and two to four ceramic teacups (unless it's imported from Japan, as I explain below). You can buy a set with matching patterns, or you might prefer to buy each item separately, mixing textures and patterns to your own taste.

Japanese teacups do not have a handle. You use both hands

to pick up a cup; one on the side, the other at the bottom. Some come with lids to keep the tea warm. Some come with saucers, which may be made of wood or lacquerware, or plastic that has been simulated to look like lacquerware. Some cups are cylinder-shaped and some bowl-shaped.

You can find Japanese or Asian-inspired teapots and cups at gourmet food and tea and coffee specialty stores like Dean & Deluca and Ito-En; at home decor and gift specialty stores like Crate & Barrel, Pottery Barn, ABC Carpet & Home, and the Museum of Modern Art Design Store; at department stores like Macy's, Neiman Marcus, and Takashimaya New York; at Japanese antique stores; and at home furnishings superstores like Bed Bath & Beyond.

An Internet search for "Japanese tea set" or "Japanese teapot" will take you to many sites that sell Japanese teaware online, like thefragrantleaf.com and yuzumura.com. Tea sets imported from Japan usually have two or five cups in a set, unlike Western sets, which typically come with four.

Easy Teaware Alternative: Use Western-style teacups and pots

Instead of an authentic Japanese tea set, you can use a teapot and the mugs and cups you already use for coffee or tea. If you are a drinker of black tea, however, it's a good idea to have a separate teapot just for green tea, so that the flavors of the two kinds of tea don't blend during the brewing.

Bowls and Plates for Japanese-Style Place Setting: How to Unlock the Magic of Japanese Portion Control

I'll tell you the secret of Japanese portion control—lots of beautiful plates and bowls, which are small enough to ensure that the servings will be small, too. And as my mother always says, "You should never fill up a bowl or plate."

In Japan, we don't combine different foods on one plate as is usually done in the West: typically a separate bowl or plate is used for each different kind of food. So when my mother makes three side dishes, everyone at the table gets three small plates or bowls, in addition to a rice bowl and a soup bowl.

What all these plates and bowls have in common is that they're much smaller than their American counterparts. And unlike Western-style tableware, Japanese plates and bowls do not all match one another, but are selected to complement the food served inside.

It is really striking how much less Billy and I started to eat when we began using Japanese plates and bowls at our apartment in New York. Since each plate is so small, we may end up helping ourselves not only to seconds, but thirds. But three servings of a very small portion is still less than one huge portion. And eating one small portion at a time helps you slow down, savor each bite, and achieve *Hara hachi bunme* ("Eat until you are 80 percent full").

For basic place settings for each person, a typical Japanese household has the following:

Rectangular and square plates are often used on Japanese tables, mainly to serve fish. I used to bring them from Japan as souvenirs for friends in America, because they were rare here and they were everywhere in Japan. Now square dishes are everywhere in America too!

Japanese rice bowls are typically ceramic with pretty patterns on the outside and often come with a matching lid. The bowls are about 4 to 5 inches in diameter and 2 to 3 inches deep, with a ½-inch rim at the bottom.

Japanese soup bowls are lacquered and often come with a matching lid, to keep the soup hot. You can find plastic ones that look like lacquerware and can go into the dishwasher for easy maintenance. The bowls are about 4 to 5 inches in diameter and 2 to 3 inches deep.

Japanese side dishes come in several sizes, and for each person there may be two to three dishes that are 3 to 5 inches in diameter, two or three bowls 3 to 5 inches in diameter and 1 to 3 inches deep, in addition to two of the square or rectangular plates typically used for fish.

Condiment plates are 2 to 3 inches in diameter. Many of the Tokyo kitchen recipes call for condiments, which are served in very small quantities on such plates. A couple of condiment plates for each person should do.

Hot noodle bowls are usually ceramic, decorated in different colors and patterns, and 5 to 6 inches in diameter and 3 to 4 inches deep.

Cold noodle trays are 6- to 7-inch-square bamboo, lacquerware, or wooden frames that are about 2 inches high, with a removable bamboo-strip strainer inside, which allows the noodles to drain.

Cold noodle dipping sauce cups are 3 to 4 inches in diameter and 2 to 3 inches high. They are typically cylindrical rather than round and are made of ceramic.

Chopsticks, of course, are the norm in all Japanese households. Just as with teacups, everyone in Japan has his or her own set of chopsticks for everyday use. Chopsticks can be made of bamboo or wood, and some are lacquered in black or red with simple pretty patterns at one end. Women's chopsticks are shorter than men's, and children's are even shorter than women's, to accommodate different hand sizes. My husband and I have matching sets in the same pattern, but the pattern on his appears against a background of black lacquer, mine on a background of red. Our names are engraved in gold—a beautiful gift from a friend of ours. We also have several sets of chopsticks for guests.

Chopstick rests are typically decorative ceramic pieces 1½ to 2 inches long and ½ to ¾ inch wide. They come in different shapes and patterns. Some are simply little colored rectangles, others are made to look like fish, vegetables, or flowers. They are used as little perches for your chopsticks, and to add pretty accents to the table.

In addition to the many small, individual-size bowls and plates, the Japanese use **serving plates, bowls, and platters** that are similar in size to those used in the West, placing them at the center of the table so that people can help themselves. They also put a ceramic or earthenware **soy sauce cruet** and **sauce-serving pitchers** in the center of the table.

Today, beautifully designed Japanese-style and Asia-inspired bowls, plates, and chopsticks are available at affordable prices at many different mainstream stores. More expensive, exquisite offerings can be found at home decor specialty stores like ABC Carpet & Home, department stores like Takashimaya New York and Barney's New York, and from brands like Casa Armani, driade, and Alessi. Products made for the U.S. market are more likely to be dishwasher- and microwave-safe than those made for Japan.

It has been said of Japanese food that it is a cuisine to be looked at rather than eaten. I would go further and say it is to be meditated upon, a kind of silent music evoked by the combination of lacquerware and the light of a candle flickering in the dark.

—Junichiro Tanizaki,
In Praise of Shadows

The only products that don't seem to be widely sold in North America are cold noodle trays and noodle sauce cups. So your best bet for finding them may be to go online. Go to e-commerce sites like www.buy4asianlife.com, www.ekitron.com, and Amazon and search with key phrases like "soba set" and "soba tray."

Easy Tableware Alternative: Use the small plates and bowls that are already on your shelves.

I really suggest you go shopping for your own set of authentic Japanese tableware. I think you'll enjoy creating a beautiful presentation with them. But in the meantime, you can improvise by using the tableware you already have.

Instead of the many specialized dishes and bowls that I described above, look in your cupboard and you'll find many possible substitutes.

Small bowls such as those used for cereal, ice cream, and soup, for example, are perfect for serving rice, miso soup, and side dishes served in a liquid. A 4-inch salad plate is perfect for stir-fried vegetables or small chunks of chilled tofu with garnish on top. A 2-inch-diameter olive dish or appetizer plate would be great for condiments like chopped scallions, or for ground white sesame seeds.

For soy sauce, you can use a creamer or an oil/vinegar cruet. For a dipping sauce pitcher, if a creamer is too small, use a gravy boat.

Hot noodles can be served in medium-size deep bowls. Cold noodles can be served in glass bowls or plates, and the accompanying dipping sauce in small bowls.

A Special Announcement: The Chopsticks Choice

I have found that using chopsticks with the finely chopped ingredients typical of Japanese home cooking helps you to eat slowly. You can pick up only so much food with these two narrow sticks, almost always much less than a mouthful.

Eating slowly is healthy, and is another way of helping you achieve the concept of *Hara hachi bunme* ("Eat until you are 80 percent full") because it allows your brain to keep pace with your stomach. When you eat quickly, the signals from the brain that tell you when you've had enough lag behind your consumption, so that by the time you know you're full, you've already eaten too much.

When you eat slowly, however, you know when you're getting full, and you can stop yourself before you're overstuffed.

Chopsticks aren't really that hard to master, and they're fun to use once you get the hang of them. And home chopsticks practice can really pay off when you go out to a Japanese, Chinese, or Korean restaurant.

But unless you're a strict Japanese food purist, I see no compelling reason not to use standard Western utensils when eating Japanese food in your home if that's what you prefer.

The important thing is to have fun and enjoy the food!

STARTER FOOD PRODUCTS FOR YOUR TOKYO KITCHEN

Japanese Ingredients—Decoded and Demystified

When I squeeze inside my mother's kitchen, I am struck by how similar it looks to a reduced version of a typical Western kitchen—stove, sink, counter, cupboards, oven, microwave oven, refrigerator—yet how radically different is much of the food that comes out of it.

The secrets are revealed on closer inspection. Scattered around the place you'll find a few pieces of cookware and a number of basic ingredients and seasonings that you'll rarely find in kitchens in the West. Once you stock up on these basics, your start-up Tokyo kitchen will be almost ready for action.

As for the ingredients, you may never have heard of some of them. You may think they have weird-sounding names and a disconcertingly mysterious appearance when you look at the packages. What in the world is "kombu"? Will it bite me? When my husband asked his sister Kate if she had ever had mugicha (a delicious cold barley tea), she replied, "Is it something you have to take medicine for?"

But unusual as they may look and sound, all these foods and ingredients are in fact both easy to understand and easy to use. Beyond that, they have three other things in common: They are the basic powerhouses of the Japanese home kitchen, providing the foundation for everything that makes Japanese home-style cooking what it is. They are used by tens of millions of Japanese women, in kitchens that are probably half the size, if not less, of yours. And you're likely to find most or all of them compatible with your own tastes if you're willing to experiment a little and give them a try.

You're also likely to find many of them at a store near you. More and more gourmet and health-oriented supermarket chains like Whole Foods and Wild Oats are carrying Japanese food ingredients in their "Asian" and "ethnic" food sections. Grocery stores in Chinatown do, too, if you have one in your city. You can also check the major supermarket chains, many of which are starting to carry the most popular Japanese home style cooking items, like tofu, miso, and soy sauce. Many health food stores carry at least some Japanese ingredients too. And if your local market does not have what you want, you can use the Internet to help you shop for Japanese ingredients. Go to Google's Froogle, Yahoo Shopping, Amazon's gourmet food section, or Web sites like www.edenfoods.com, where you'll find a number of sources for Japanese goodies.

Best of all, if you're lucky enough to live near a Japanese grocery store, or an Asian, Korean, or "Oriental" specialty market that carries Japanese food items, you'll feel like you hit the jackpot since you'll be able to pick from a wide range of products, often at prices lower than what you'll find in regular supermarkets.

There are close to two hundred Japanese-focused food markets around the United States, many of them clustered in

Northern and Southern California, the greater New York area, and Hawaii. To find out if there's one near you, go to the "Yellow Pages Japan in USA" English-language Web site at www.ypj.com/en and enter the keyword "markets," then select your city and state.

If you live in Manhattan, for example, you can buy your Japanese groceries at Sunrise Mart, which has stores in both the East Village and SoHo, or JAS Mart, which has stores on Twenty-third Street in the Flatiron district and in the East Village, or Yagura Market on East Forty-first Street between Fifth and Madison Avenues, or Katagiri on East Fifty-ninth Street. Just across the Hudson River is the enormous Mitsuwa Marketplace in Edgewater, New Jersey, one of the nine branches of an extraordinarily well-stocked Japanese superstore that we are fortunate to have in the United States.

In California, you've got dozens of Japanese grocery stores to choose from, including other branches of the Mitsuwa Marketplace, branches of the Nijiya Market and Marukai chains, and independent specialty markets in Los Angeles's Little Tokyo, in nearby Orange County, and in San Francisco's Japantown. There are also Japanese markets in San Jose, San Mateo, Cupertino, Berkeley, Monterey, San Diego, Torrance, Sacramento, and a number of other California cities.

But it's not just California, New York, and Hawaii—you'll also find Japanese grocery stores in Arizona, Oregon, Florida, Georgia, Ohio, and Illinois. Kentucky has one: the Hibari Market on Redding Drive in Lexington. In Pittsburgh, you can check out the Tokyo Japanese Food Store on Ellsworth Avenue. You can even find a Japanese market in Indianapolis:

Sakura Mart, on Seventy-first Street on the north side of town.

When shopping in an ethnic market, the main thing is not to let yourself be intimidated by how foreign-looking the products are. Since Japanese grocery stores stock seasonings and ingredients imported from Japan, the packaging is also directly from Japan, which means that most of the writing is in Japanese. Not to worry. On the back of almost every product is a label in English, listing the product name, ingredients, nutrition facts, manufacturer, and importer. And don't get overwhelmed by the sheer abundance of what you see on the shelves. Keep in mind that just like bread or milk in this country, each of the basic Japanese food ingredients and seasonings comes in many different varieties from many different manufacturers. In fact, you may at first think there are too many. Having such an array of choices can be very confusing.

I know the feeling. I was once a Japanese girl fresh off the plane and newly transplanted to the bewilderingly vast consumer culture of America; I felt lost every time I walked into a supermarket. Just to buy milk, I had to choose among whole milk, skim, low-fat (1% or 2%), half and half, lactose-free, soy, rice, in different sizes—not to mention having to choose which brand I preferred. This was completely overwhelming to me. I was terrified to go food shopping.

Which reminds me of a man I know named Mel Berger.

He is one of the top literary agents in New York. In fact, he is my agent. He is a deal maker. I've seen him in action in business, and he comes across as brilliant and fearless. But this man Mel Berger has a secret fear.

He lives in New Jersey, close to a branch of that fantastic Japanese grocery store—the Mitsuwa Marketplace. Inside its doors is a wonderland of Japanese home cooking ingredients and equipment, foods, beverages, flavorings, cakes and sweets, fresh vegetables and succulent fruit, some of it fresh off the plane from Tokyo.

Mel likes Japanese food. Yet he has never gone inside. Why?

"Because," he confessed to me quietly one day, "I'm afraid of it."

"Why are you afraid?" I asked.

He replied, "I don't know what's in it."

Although it can be intimidating to shop for products that seem foreign to you, knowledge is power, and the unfamiliar will soon become familiar. Even once you've worked up the courage to buy these ingredients, however, some may seem a bit strange to your taste. Don't give up on the first trial tasting, just because you or a family member did not like the flavor. Try small tastes of many different dishes, until you find the ones you like. And don't decide on the basis of any one tasting that you don't like a whole category of food, because within a given category there are so many different tastes.

Take miso, for example. For the Japanese, miso is like wine, cheese, or coffee to you—something very familiar that comes in dozens of subtle varieties of flavor, aroma, color, and texture. As you'll read below, some misos are mild and sweet, others salty and pungent; some are smooth and refined, others slightly coarse or pebbly in texture. You might love one kind of miso and not another.

You will probably not know what style of miso you prefer. But how did you find out which blend and brand of coffee you like most? Did you stick with the first you tried, or switch among several until you found your current favorite? And what about wine? If you're a wine lover, I'm sure you have your standbys, but you probably are always learning about new wines to enjoy. Apply a similar process to researching your favorites when you shop for your Tokyo kitchen. Testing and tasting is part of the pleasure of cooking and eating.

That's what I discovered when I first came to America and ate cheese here. In Japan, when I was growing up, we had basically one kind of cheese. It was a processed, gooey, semihard block. Sliced into small rectangular shapes, it was layered onto slices of bread that we toasted, or it was grilled with eggs, put into salads or sandwiches, or eaten plain. This was all I knew of cheese, and no matter how we used it, I never found its taste or texture appealing.

Only in America did I become acquainted with the wonderful world of cheese. In Illinois, I was introduced to the famous cheeses of nearby Wisconsin. Now I love to eat wedges of those sharp tangy cheeses with slices of apple. And I've learned about lots of other cheeses since then. I break and sprinkle Roquefort cheese with dried cranberries over salad. I smear goat cheese from my local farmers market on thinly sliced baguettes I buy at a great bakery in my neighborhood. And I love to prepare a simple dish of fresh mozzarella with ripe tomato slices sprinkled with olive oil and fresh basil. So, never say never!

Tokyo Kitchen Key Ingredients

The shopping list on page 121 will help you get started on your Tokyo kitchen. Take it with you the first few times you go shopping for Japanese ingredients. Almost all the items on the list, with the exception of tofu and daikon radish, will keep for weeks to months on a shelf or in the refrigerator, and are the kinds of things that a typical Tokyo kitchen always has on hand for daily use.

These are the staples, the basics. Of course you'll also be shopping for fresh foods as needed.

Here is an introduction to the items on your new Tokyo kitchen shopping list.

BONITO (FISH) FLAKES (Katsuobushi, Hana-katsuo, or Kezuri-bushi)

A member of the mackerel family, bonito generally makes its appearance in Japanese cuisine not as a whole fish but as dried bonito fish flakes. These fish flakes or katsuobushi are an important ingredient in the Japanese kitchen. The large fish flakes are used to make dashi, the essential cooking stock (page 52), while the smaller flakes are used as a garnish for many dishes.

Bonito flakes look like paper-thin curls of wood and range in color from pinky beige to dark burgundy. Although many Japanese make their own fish flakes with a special bonito shaving implement, you can buy commercially shaved flakes in clear plastic bags. Large flakes for making dashi range in quantity from 1- to 16-ounce bags. The small fish flakes typically used for garnishes come in single-serving packets, usually five to a bag, with individual packets weighing anywhere from 0.52 to 0.88 ounces.

Bonito flakes have a mild, smoky, faintly sweet flavor. Although it's probably unlike anything you've encountered in Western cooking, it's an easy-to-like taste.

DAIKON (Japanese Giant White Radish)

Daikon is a large white Japanese radish. It is quite juicy and has a fresh, sweet flavor and a mild bite. In her book *An American Taste of Japan*, Tokyo-based writer Elizabeth Andoh, the dean of Western authorities on Japanese food, notes that daikon "is perhaps the single most versatile vegetable in the Japanese repertoire; it can be grated or shredded and eaten raw; it can be steamed or braised and sauced or included in stews; it can be pickled or dried, too."

I particularly like serving raw grated daikon with oily foods, since the spicy, wet radish provides an ideal counterpoint to deep-fried items and fatty fish, much the way lemon does in Western cooking. Daikon also makes a tasty addition to miso soup—turning soft and almost sweet as it simmers in the savory liquid.

Several varieties of fresh daikon are available in the United States, including a green-necked version, which has a pale collar of green around the stem top area. When buying daikon, choose ones that are firm, not limp.

Snap Peas, Daikon, and Egg Soup

SERVES 4

This is one of my favorite dishes from my mother's Tokyo kitchen. Growing up, I often had it for breakfast, accompanied by thick slices of toast and two or more little side dishes. It is my mother's original creation. The flavor from this soup comes primarily from the wok-sizzled egg, which has a rich toasty browned flavor. I love biting into the egg chunks, tasting the distinct green, earthy flavors of the snap peas and scallion mingled with the sweet, tender flavor of the yellow onion, and sipping the soup, its complex layering of flavors all blending into one. It tastes gorgeous—so light and so satisfying at the same time!

4 large eggs

2 scallions, roots and tops cut off

3 tablespoons canola oil or rice bran oil

2/3 cup finely diced yellow onion (about 1/2 medium onion)

2/3 cup finely diced peeled daikon

1 shiitake mushroom, stem cut off, cap finely sliced

5 cups dashi (page 52)

1 teaspoon sake

1 teaspoon fine-ground sea salt

Freshly ground black pepper

20 snap peas (or snow peas), strings removed, each pea
    diagonally cut into thirds

1 teaspoon reduced-sodium soy sauce

1. Break the eggs into a medium bowl and whisk until thoroughly mixed.
2. Cut one of the scallions into half-inch long batons for the soup. Thinly slice the other scallion to use as a garnish.
3. Place a wok (or a large skillet with good heat conductivity) over high heat. Add 2 tablespoons of the oil and swirl it around to coat the interior of the wok. When the oil begins to simmer, lower the heat to medium-high and add the beaten eggs; they will form a disc and immediately begin to puff and bubble around the edges. Fry the egg disc for 2 minutes, or until the center portion is no longer runny. Turn the egg disc and fry for 1 more minute. Transfer to a plate. When the egg disc is cool enough to handle, tear it into bite-size pieces.
4. Add the remaining 1 tablespoon of oil to the wok. When hot, add the onion, daikon, and mushroom. Stir-fry for 3 minutes. Add the dashi, sake, salt, and several grinds of pepper, and bring to a boil. Skim off foam on the surface with a ladle. Reduce the heat to medium and simmer the soup for about 3 minutes, or until the daikon has turned translucent.
6. Add the bits of torn omelette to the soup, along with the snap peas, scallion batons, and soy. Cook over high heat for 1 to 2 minutes, or until the snap peas are crisp-tender.
7. Lay out 4 large soup bowls and ladle equal portions of the soup into them. Garnish with the thinly sliced scallion.

JAPANESE-STYLE SHORT-GRAIN RICE

Short-grain white rice is standard for Japanese home cooking. It is moister and stickier than medium- and long-grain rice. Short-grain brown rice, or genmai, is a high-fiber alternative.

Personally, I like to switch between white rice, brown rice, and a third interesting option, haiga-mai (literally, rice-germ rice). This rice is partially polished, so it still contains the nutritious rice germ (usually removed in the milling process). I find haiga-mai tastes more nutty than polished white rice, but not quite as hearty as brown. Unlike the other rice types, haiga-mai should not be rinsed before cooking, in order to preserve the germ.

A premium variety of short-grain rice popular among Japanese is Koshihikari. Traditionally grown in Japan, and sold under a number of different brand labels, this sweet, aromatic rice is now cultivated in the United States too.

In my opinion, American-grown short-grain rice is just as tasty as Japanese-grown rice and often less expensive. Some rice brands I like include Kagayaki, Kokuho Rose, Tamaki, and Lundberg Family Farms, all of which are grown in the United States.

Store all rice in an airtight container in a cool, dry place, for up to a year.

JAPANESE TEAS

Green Teas

From sunrise to sundown, green tea flows like water in most Japanese homes and restaurants. And although the Japanese love coffee and black tea, they're crazy about their green tea.

It seems like there's green tea brewing in my parents' dining room or kitchen all day long. When I'm there, my mother never asks, "Would you like some tea?" She just keeps pouring it.

Japanese green tea is gentle and clean-tasting, almost the opposite of coffee. It rejuvenates the soul, refreshes the palate, and heals the body. Ancient priests and poets throughout China and Japan, as well as contemporary Western health experts, such as Andrew Weil, have sung the praises of this antioxidant superstar.

Green tea is *never* served with sugar or cream, unless it becomes an ingredient for a dessert like green tea ice cream.

There are many varieties of green tea. Here are descriptions of some of the most popular:

Sencha is the most popular green tea in a traditional Japanese home. It is grown in the sun.

Gyokuro, grown in the shade, is the finest, most expensive Japanese green tea.

Shin cha, or new tea, is freshly harvested green tea, available in early summer.

Hojicha is roasted green tea leaves. When brewed, the tea, like the leaves themselves, is brown. It has a milder flavor than sencha, and makes a great companion to fruits and other desserts.

Genmaicha is a mixture of green tea leaves and roasted brown rice. The rice adds a nutty, sweet grainy flavor to the tea.

Genmaimatcha is a mixture of green tea leaves, roasted brown rice, and powdered green tea. It has layers of flavor, and is one of my favorites.

Barley Tea

Mugicha (pronounced "moo-*gee*-cha") is barley tea. Made cold, it is a healthy and delicious summertime drink; all year-round, it's a great substitute for the sweetened and carbonated beverages Westerners favor.

Tea Leaves, Tea Bags, and Bottles

As with black tea, Japanese green tea is available in many forms: loose leaves, in tea bags, and ready to drink in a bottle. With the exception of barley tea, I prefer to make my tea with loose leaves instead of bags because the leaves create a more fragrant and flavorful brew.

In the United States, you can find high-quality Japanese green tea leaves at tea specialty stores like Peet's Coffee & Tea, Harney & Sons Master Tea Blenders, and Ito-En; at department stores like Takashimaya New York; and at Japanese grocery stores.

For ready-to-drink Japanese teas, one of my favorite brands is Teas' Tea, made by the Japanese tea company Ito-En. Teas' Tea offers a tasty selection of cold and hot teas that can be found in many delis and supermarkets.

MIRIN (Cooking Wine)

Mirin is a sweet, golden cooking wine, made from glutenous rice, that has an alcohol content of about 14 percent. It comes in a bottle and is used in many Japanese home-style recipes to add a bit of sweetness to simmered dishes, glazes, and sauces.

MISO (Fermented Soybean Paste)

Miso is a thick, salty fermented soybean paste that looks something like peanut butter and comes in refrigerated pouches or plastic tubs.

It is made from crushed soybeans, salt, a fermenting agent, and the addition of barley, rice, or wheat. Depending upon which grain is added, the miso will vary tremendously in flavor, texture, aroma, and color. Miso can range in flavor from salty to sweet; in texture from smooth to slightly pebbly to chunky (with the addition of crushed grains or soybeans); in smell from delicate to pungent; and in color from beige to golden yellow to brown.

In its many variations, miso is a staple of the Japanese kitchen and adds a savory base note to soups, dressings, simmered dishes, and stir-fries.

So-called white miso is actually pale yellow and has a milder, sweeter flavor than other miso varieties. Because of its delicate nature, it's often used for dressings (particularly for vegetables) and in marinades for mild-tasting fish and seafood.

So-called red miso, which appears rusty brown, is coarser and saltier than white. It works best in marinades and sauces for meats. The darkest brown version of red miso has the sharpest flavor and tastes best when added to simmered dishes containing oily fish or hearty meats. There are also mixed red-and-white versions of miso.

For miso soup as well as other dishes, many Japanese cooks keep two or three different kinds of miso in the refrigerator so that they can combine them to achieve their preferred taste.

Like soy sauce, miso can sometimes be very high in salt, so look for lower-sodium or reduced-sodium miso by carefully reading labels.

Miso brands I particularly like include Miso Master from American Miso Company and Westbrae.

Restaurant chefs around the world have discovered the magic of miso and are using this bean paste to add a savory flavor boost to a variety of dishes—not just Asian ones.

Store miso in an airtight container in a refrigerator.

Eggplant Sautéed with Miso

SERVES 4

Japanese eggplants come in a variety of sizes and shapes. However, they are much smaller than the football-shaped ones sold in American markets. What's more, they have firmer and sweeter flesh. For this recipe, try to find four 4-inch-long eggplants, which are typically considered medium size in Japan.

The thick miso sauce in this eggplant dish has a delightful sweet-savory tang that my husband, Billy, likens to a Japanese-style barbecue sauce.

> 1 pound Japanese eggplants (or Italian eggplants), stem
> caps cut off, cut into bite-size pieces
>
> 2 tablespoons mirin
>
> 2 tablespoons red miso
>
> 2 teaspoons granulated sugar
>
> 1 teaspoon sake
>
> 1 cup canola oil or rice bran oil
>
> 1 green bell pepper, cored, seeded, and cut into bite-
> size pieces
>
> 1 teaspoon toasted and ground white sesame seeds
>
> 1/2 teaspoon toasted sesame oil

1. Soak the cut eggplant pieces in a bowl of water for a few minutes. Drain water and thoroughly wipe and blot the eggplant with paper towels.

2. In a small bowl, blend the mirin, miso, sugar, and sake. Set aside.

3. Heat the oil in a wok or large deep skillet over medium heat until it reaches 350°F. If you don't have a thermometer, test the oil with a tiny square of fresh bread (or a piece of panko). If the bread rises and immediately turns golden, then the oil is hot enough. Slip the eggplant pieces, one of the flesh sides down, into the oil. Fry for 3 minutes, adjusting the heat as necessary to keep the oil temperature around 350°F. Rotate and fry the eggplant on all sides for 1 to 2 minutes more, or until the flesh is soft. Test for doneness by piercing the flesh with a wooden skewer: you should be able to slide it easily all the way through. Transfer the eggplant pieces to a rack lined with a double layer of paper towels and place them cut side down to drain.

4. Pour off the oil from the wok into a metal container (to discard or use on another occasion). The wok will still be coated with a small amount of oil. Place the wok over medium-high heat and add the pepper. Stir-fry for 2 minutes, or until the pepper is bright green. Add the eggplant pieces and the miso mixture and gently toss the vegetables to coat with the sauce. Transfer to a serving dish and garnish with the toasted and ground sesame seeds and sesame oil.

NOODLES

Japan is awash in noodles. Family noodle shops dot the entire country from the northern island of Hokkaido to the Ryukyu Islands south of Kyushu. My mother loves to make a variety of noodle dishes and so do I. Some of the best meals I've eaten in Japan (aside from Mom's cooking, of course!) have come from nondescript mom-and-pop noodle shops. Whenever I go home to Tokyo, the first meal I have off the plane is almost always a bowl of noodles.

Japanese noodles fall into two major camps: those made with buckwheat flour (soba), and those made with white wheat flour (udon).

Egg noodles, or ramen, are also very popular in Japan, mostly enjoyed as packaged instant soups or in ramen specialty shops.

Soba (Buckwheat Noodles)

Soba is the name for noodles made from buckwheat flour. They are thin, grayish brown, and delightfully nutty tasting with a silky smooth texture. They are served hot in soups, as well as cold with a tasty sweet soy dipping sauce (see pages 200 and 202 for hot and cold soba noodle recipes).

Because buckwheat flour lacks gluten, the component in wheat flour that gives noodles their pleasant chew, most noodle makers add a little bit of starch to the dough. Some soba manufacturers add too much starch (in the form of white wheat flour or yam flour)—mainly to cut costs, since buckwheat flour costs more than other flours. The result is an inferior soba noodle that lacks the distinctive earthy flavor.

Look for noodles that are as close to 100 percent buckwheat as possible. Soba noodles made exclusively from buckwheat flour are really worth the search. Brands like Eden Foods, for example, sell them online. Among soba purists, these dark brown noodles are considered the best.

Udon and Other White Flour Noodles

One of the most popular kinds of white flour noodle is udon. They are thick and white and have a wonderful chewy texture. They are eaten hot in soups with a variety of toppings or cold with dipping sauce.

Other tasty white flour noodles you might encounter include kishimen, which are chewy, flat, and wide, almost like fettuccine. Somen is a snow white noodle as thin as angel hair and almost always served cold in the summer. A slightly thicker version of somen is hiyamugi.

———

As with Italian pasta, I think fresh noodles taste the best. Throughout Japan, trained noodle masters sell handmade soba and udon from their shops. However, since it's hard to find fresh soba and udon in the West, all the noodle recipes in my Tokyo kitchen call for dried noodles. But don't worry, high-quality dried soba and udon are readily available and very tasty!

OILS

Canola Oil

Canola oil is one of the best vegetable oils to cook with, because it has among the highest concentrations of the good fats—polyunsaturated fat and monounsaturated fat—and the lowest of the bad kind of fat—saturated fat. And except in its hydrogenated form, it has absolutely none of the worst fat of all—trans fat. Because canola oil has little flavor, I find it allows the pure natural flavor of ingredients to shine through. For these reasons, I have called for it in all of my Tokyo kitchen recipes, whenever a cooking oil is used.

In Tokyo, my mother uses canola oil for almost all of her frying and sautéing. She occasionally uses olive oil for Western dishes, which can handle the strong flavor of the oil, but olive oil is too overpowering for Japanese food.

Look for *nonhydrogenated* canola oil.

Rice Bran Oil

Rice bran oil is an extremely light, delicate oil expressed from the outer grain hull of rice. It is great for stir-frying and sautéing. I find it lighter than canola oil and it, too, has virtually no flavor. It is also high in good fats like polyunsaturated fat and monounsaturated fat, making it another ideal healthy cooking oil for your Tokyo kitchen.

However, it is not widely available in supermarkets. If you want to try it, hunt for it online or at a Japanese grocery store.

Sesame Oil

Extracted from sesame seeds, sesame oil comes in two types: light and dark (also called toasted). The lighter oil has a softer flavor and color than the dark version. Its potent flavor makes it appropriate to use as a garnish. My mother likes to drizzle dark sesame oil over hot-cooked foods because she finds the heat intensifies the oil's nutty flavor and aroma.

Sesame oil can be used as cooking oil, but I seldom do since it burns too fast for my taste. Instead, I sprinkle it on stir-fried vegetables as soon as I turn off the heat, and use it in my salad dressings (see page 167 for a recipe).

RICE VINEGAR

In addition to the fried, steamed, and simmered categories of Japanese cooking, there is a fourth category: "vinegared" dishes, typically served as appetizers or side dishes. The rice vinegar used in these dishes is made either from white rice or brown rice. Regular rice vinegar ranges in color from light to golden yellow, while brown rice vinegar ranges from brown to black. Brown rice vinegar tastes milder than regular rice vinegar—yet rice vinegar overall has much less of a bite than pungent Western vinegars. Even when I'm making Western-style salads, I prefer to make my dressings with rice vinegar, since it's not as sour as white or red vinegar. If you have ever eaten sushi, you are already familiar with the taste of rice vinegar, since the sushi rice is gently tossed with a mixture of rice vinegar, sugar, and salt.

RICE WINE (Sake)

Sake, which is made from fermented rice grains, not only makes a delightful alcoholic drink but also adds an indispensable touch to many Japanese dishes. Sake adds depth to simmered dishes, sauces, and dressings, and it reduces fish and meat odors. In my mother's Tokyo kitchen, a small amount of sake is used to help balance out the sweet and savory flavors in many of her recipes.

Sake comes in numerous styles and, like wine, ranges enormously in quality, price, and flavor, from dry to quite sweet. My mother favors good-quality sake when it comes to cooking. Just as most good Western cooks avoid "cooking wine," she eschews inexpensive so-called cooking sake because it contains added ingredients like sugar and salt that she feels detract from rather than enhance her food.

Since the alcohol in sake evaporates during cooking, you can still cook with it even if you avoid alcohol.

SEA VEGETABLES (Seaweed)

Sea vegetables play an integral role in the Japanese diet. They are nutritious, tasty, and extremely versatile. They flavor stocks, are found in cold salads, and add a savory crunch to rice and noodle dishes.

Hijiki

Hijiki is a dark seaweed that comes in thin, dry, ribbonlike strands and is the basis for many popular home-style dishes. When freshly harvested, hijiki is reddish brown. After it is steamed and dried, it turns almost black, which is how it is sold. Before hijiki can be cooked, it must be reconstituted in cold water.

Kombu

Kombu, also known as konbu or kobu, is considered the king of seaweeds in Japan. A kind of kelp, it is thick, leafy, and brownish green. Outside of Japan, kombu is primarily available dried, often in rectangles from 1 x 5 inches to 5 x 10 inches for dashi.

When steeped in water with dried bonito flakes, kombu makes the clear cooking stock dashi (see page 52), used as a basis for so many Japanese dishes. It's also enjoyed simmered (as an accompaniment to white rice) and dried as a snack.

Nori

Often called "laver" outside of Japan, nori refers to the thin, flat sheets of dried seaweed that range in color from pine green to purple black. If you've ever eaten sushi rolls, you've tasted nori. It's the crackly dark green substance that wraps around the vinegared rice (and eventually becomes soft and slightly chewy the longer it sits).

A popular Japanese snack that uses nori is onigiri, or rice

balls. Every convenience store in Japan has a section devoted to these small vegetable- or fish-stuffed rice balls (or triangles) sealed with nori (see page 176 for a recipe).

Nori used to make sushi is often toasted and comes labeled "Sushi Nori." Toasting enhances the flavor and crisp texture of the seaweed. Sushi nori usually comes in large 8-inch squares with several sheets to a bag. Because nori loses its crispness as soon as it is exposed to air, remove only one sheet at a time for whatever you're making and keep the bag sealed at all times. To store, place the nori in an airtight container or zip-top bag.

Shredded nori makes a popular garnish for rice and noodle dishes. You can buy containers of commercially cut nori, or make your own, cutting a sheet of nori into a pile of ⅛ x 1-inch strips (or squares, as I sometimes do).

Seasoned nori sheets are also available. The crisp sheets are brushed with a sweet soy-based sauce and often sold in small rectangles with only a few sheets to each package. Seasoned nori sheets wrapped around hot cooked rice are a popular Japanese breakfast treat, and so easy to make. You simply take a small sheet of seasoned nori and quickly dip one side in some soy sauce. Then wrap the seaweed around a mouthful of rice from your rice bowl. Alternatively, tear the seasoned nori into small bits and scatter them over your rice.

Hijiki Sea Vegetable and Fried Tofu

SERVES 4

Although the recipe calls for a very small amount of dried hijiki, don't worry that you won't have enough. This nutritious sea vegetable, or seaweed, which looks like very small black pasta, expands both during soaking and cooking. Hijiki has a crisp-soft texture and an earthy flavor. Soft meaty tofu slices and dashi-based simmering sauce complement the hijiki, making a small yet dramatic side dish.

1/4 cup dried hijiki (sea vegetable)
1/2 of a 3-x-5-inch rectangle of usu-age tofu (thin fried
   tofu)
2/3 cup dashi (page 52)
1 tablespoon sake
1 tablespoon mirin
2 1/2 teaspoons reduced-sodium soy sauce
1 teaspoon granulated sugar
1/4 teaspoon salt
1 1/2 teaspoons canola oil or rice bran oil

1. Rinse the hijiki in a bowl of cold water, and drain it over a fine mesh strainer.
2. Soak the rinsed hijiki in lukewarm water, according to the package directions, until tender, about 30 minutes. Drain.

3. Bring a small saucepan of water to a boil. Add the half portion of usu-age tofu and gently simmer over medium heat, turning occasionally, for 1 minute; drain (this will remove excess oil). Cut the tofu diagonally in half and slice each half into thin strips.

4. Combine the dashi, sake, mirin, soy, sugar, and salt in a small bowl. Whisk until the sugar has dissolved.

5. Heat the oil in a medium nonstick skillet over medium heat. When hot, add the hijiki and sauté for 5 minutes. Stir in the fried tofu strips.

6. Add the dashi mixture, reduce the heat to medium-low, and simmer for 12 to 15 minutes, or until the liquid has evaporated. The hijiki will swell as it cooks and absorb the seasoning mix. Transfer to a small serving dish.

SESAME SEEDS (goma)

In Japanese home cooking, white and black sesame seeds add a fragrant nutty accent to all kinds of dishes. I recommend buying untoasted whole sesame seeds. Toasting the seeds right before use brings out their buttery richness. The seeds are used to garnish vegetable, tofu, seafood, and meat dishes, as well as to flavor dipping sauces.

Grinding the seeds turns them into a flaky base used for dressings and sauces. Most Japanese cooks grind their sesame seeds with a wooden mortar in a ribbed ceramic bowl called a suribachi. You can grind them in a food processor, or with a mortar and pestle. Or you can buy sesame seeds already ground. But I prefer to grind sesame seeds myself immediately before using them, for heightened aroma and flavor.

Toasted and Ground White Sesame Seeds

¼ cup whole white sesame seeds

1. To toast the sesame seeds, place them in a medium dry saucepan over medium heat. Move the pan in a circular motion, approximately 1 inch above the flame (or heating coil), so that the seeds continually swirl around the bottom of the pan. Continue toasting the seeds in this manner until they begin to turn shiny and honey colored, about 6 minutes. Watch the seeds carefully, as they brown quickly toward the end of cooking. Immediately remove the pan from the heat and transfer the seeds to a bowl to prevent them from over-cooking.

2. To grind the toasted sesame seeds, place them in a food processor with a metal blade and process until they are just coarsely chopped (too much processing will turn them into sesame paste). Alternatively, place the seeds in a mortar with a pestle and grind them until flaky. Or lay a large square of cheesecloth on a wooden cutting board. Place the toasted sesame seeds in the center of the cloth and fold the cloth in half, gently pushing the seeds around to distribute them even-ly. Using a large knife, "chop" the seeds through the cloth. The knife will not cut through the cheesecloth, but instead crush the seeds to a flaky consistency.

SHISO

Shiso is an herb in the mint family. Quite fragrant with a slightly bitter, mintlike flavor, shiso leaves are about 2 inches square, heart-shaped with jagged edges. Shiso grows in green and reddish purple color varieties. Whole shiso leaves are commonly used in Japan as a garnish for sashimi, and as an ingredient in tempura. Finely chopped leaves are used as a seasoning for tofu and other dishes, and the dried chopped red leaves can be sprinkled on hot rice for flavoring. In early summer, pale pink shiso flowers on a short stem are used as a decorative and edible seasonal garnish. All shiso leaves used in my Tokyo kitchen recipes are the green and fresh kind. You can find them at Asian and Japanese grocers, gourmet marketplaces, and green markets.

Tokyo Fried Chicken

SERVES 4

Despite being fried, these gingery nuggets of chicken are crisp and greaseless. The trick to successful deep-frying lies in using hot, clean oil, and frying only a handful of items at the same time (to avoid overcrowding and cooling down the oil, which results in soggy, grease-laden food—the opposite of what you want). Shredded shiso is a perfect counterpoint to the chicken because its peppery freshness offsets the chicken's fried coating.

4 boneless, skinless chicken breasts (4 to 6 ounces each),
   cut into bite-size pieces
One 2-inch-long chunk fresh ginger
1 tablespoon reduced-sodium soy sauce
2 teaspoons sake
1 teaspoon mirin
½ cup katakuriko (potato starch) or cornstarch
About 2 cups canola oil or rice bran oil, for deep-frying
4 shiso leaves, for garnish, cut into very thin ribbons
Reduced-sodium soy sauce, to use at the table

1. Place the chicken in a medium bowl.
2. Line a small bowl with cheesecloth. Grate the ginger over the bowl, gather the cheesecloth around the ginger, and squeeze the cheesecloth over the bowl to release the ginger juice. You should have approximately 1½ teaspoons of ginger juice. Pour the ginger juice over the chicken, along with the soy, sake, and mirin. Toss the chicken to coat and let marinate for 10 minutes.
3. Place the katakuriko (or cornstarch) in a small bowl. Remove the chicken from the marinade and blot any excess marinade from the chicken with paper towels. Working with a few pieces of chicken at a time, drop them into the starch and push them around until well coated. Transfer the dredged chicken pieces to a platter.
4. Heat the oil in a wok or large deep skillet over medium heat until it reaches 350°F. If you don't have a thermometer, test the oil with a pinch of flour. If the flour rises to the surface of the oil and immediately turns golden, then the oil is hot enough. Working in batches, add one third of the chicken to the oil. Fry

for 1 minute on each side (adjusting the heat as necessary to keep the oil temperature around 350°F), or until the chicken is golden and just cooked through. (Test a piece by removing it from the oil and cutting it in half.) Transfer the fried chicken to a platter lined with a double layer of paper towels. Bring the temperature of the oil back to 350°F and cook the remaining two batches of chicken in the same manner.

5. Transfer the chicken to a large serving dish. Sprinkle it with the shiso ribbons and bring to the table, along with a bottle of soy. Let each diner season his or her own portion of chicken with soy.

SOY SAUCE (Shoyu)

Soy sauce, or shoyu, is a Japanese home-style-cooking work-horse. This dark brown liquid, derived from soybeans, barley (or wheat), salt, and water, has a distinctive savory richness that gives Japanese cooking its signature flavor. In addition to seasoning soups, sauces, marinades, and dressings, soy sauce serves as an indispensable condiment for dishes like sushi.

However, *soy sauce should be used with a delicate hand.* Many Westerners make the mistake of saturating their food with soy sauce, not realizing that a little goes a very long way. When used properly and sparingly, soy sauce should bring out, not overwhelm, the innate flavor of an ingredient.

Because regular soy sauce contains high amounts of sodium, I feel it is one of the few nonhealthy ingredients in the traditional Japanese pantry. (Some varieties of miso also suffer from the same high-sodium problem.)

However, there is a solution: use *reduced-sodium soy sauce.*

To me, reduced-sodium soy sauce tastes just as good, if not better, than regular soy sauce. Most supermarkets carry reduced-sodium soy sauce. All the Tokyo kitchen recipes in this book call for reduced-sodium soy sauce.

A high-quality wheat-free alternative to soy sauce that's popular among health food devotees and people with wheat allergies is tamari. It tastes similar to soy and also comes in reduced-sodium varieties.

TOFU

Tofu is coagulated soy milk, made from soybeans and fashioned into blocks.

Most tofu is white with a hint of light yellow, like vanilla ice cream. Unlike in the United States, where tofu hasn't yet fully outlived its reputation as a hippie-inspired, tasteless health food, tofu is extremely popular in Japan. It's a sort of meat-and-potatoes ingredient for most Japanese home cooks, including my mother, and there are hundreds of delicious ways to prepare it.

Among tofu's many merits is its high-protein content. As a result, it makes a terrific substitute for all kinds of meats, poultry, and seafood. When it's of good quality, it has a subtle, clean, lightly earthy taste.

Tofu is incredibly versatile. It can be added to appetizers, soups, main courses, dressings, and desserts, as well as eaten on its own—hot or cold—with various garnishes.

Tofu also delights the palate with its wide variety of textures, depending upon how it's prepared. Steaming, for example, turns tofu plump and juicy, while stir-frying turns it crispy, firm, and golden. When stewed, tofu becomes tender and succulent, and when whipped in a blender or food processor, it becomes creamy and thick, like sour cream.

Tofu is sold in various forms. The two basic kinds are known as "silken" and "cotton," and both may come in different degrees of firmness. Since the language used by different manufacturers to describe the several variations within those two general categories is not always consistent, here are some general directions to help you navigate through the tofu landscape.

Silken tofu, or kinugoshi tofu, is extremely delicate, with a porcelainlike color and a custard-pudding-like texture both outside and inside. This lovely texture is achieved because silken types of tofu, unlike the cotton types, are coagulated without being pressed to eliminate excess water.

For its external beauty and ever-so-subtle flavor, silken tofu is used in elegant soups, or chilled and eaten on its own with various garnishes (see pages 189 and 49).

Because silken tofu is so delicate, when my mother uses it she transfers the fragile tofu block directly from the container onto the palm of her left hand. She then uses her right hand to very carefully cut the tofu with a knife into even, bite-size or smaller pieces. She then slides them with great care onto a plate or into water or broth that is gently simmering in a saucepan. All of this gentle handling is for the purpose of making sure that the tofu remains intact in little squares, which look so pretty floating, for instance, in a clear soup. If she were to cut the silken tofu on a chopping board, some pieces might break up when they were transferred from the chopping board to the saucepan or the plate.

Silken tofu is sold in airtight plastic containers with water, or in aseptic packaging without water. The waterless packaging means that it can keep indefinitely on the shelf. The water-packed variety has a shorter shelf life and should be used as soon as opened.

Cotton (as it's known in Japan) or **firm** tofu, is less fragile than silken and, the "firm" designation notwithstanding, it comes in textures generally labeled soft, medium firm, firm, and extra firm. Generally speaking, the recipes in this book that call for cotton tofu use the firm texture, though that is more a matter of taste than necessity.

Because it's made by a different process than silken tofu, a process that involves separating the curds from the whey of the soy milk and then compressing the curds, the texture of cotton tofu is much firmer (even in its so-called soft versions). Cotton tofu has a slightly coarse surface and a much more substantial bite and texture than silken, which makes it suitable for stir-fries and for grilled and simmered dishes (see page 118). It is almost always sold in water-filled cartons.

Tofu is sold by many different manufacturers in the United States. Some brands, like Nasoya, make both silken and cotton varieties. Nasoya's silken comes only in the soft texture, while its cotton comes in soft, firm, and extra firm textures. House Foods America also makes both silken and cotton, the silken in extra soft and soft while the cotton comes in medium firm, firm, and extra firm. Mori-Nu makes only silken tofu, but its silken tofu is available as silken soft, silken firm, and silken extra firm.

Tofu is also sold fried. When fried, tofu becomes firm and takes on an appealing meatiness, thus making it a terrific addition to soups and vegetable dishes.

Thick-fried tofu rectangles (about 3-x-5-x-1 inch) are

known as **atsu-age** tofu. Thin-fried tofu rectangles (about 3-x-5-x-⅓ inches) are known as **usu-age** tofu.

Both thin- and thick-fried are golden yellow on the outside and creamy white inside. Typically, atsu-age tofu is packed in an airtight plastic bag, and usu-age in a plastic bag. In America, these are usually sold in the freezer section of Japanese markets (see pages 22, 57, 160, and 190 for recipes with atsu-age and usu-age tofu).

Yakidofu, or broiled tofu, is firm cotton tofu that has been broiled and has scorch marks on the surface. It's packed in water in a plastic container like the various kinds of cotton tofu, but tastes a tad smoky. It is used in sukiyaki dishes in Japan.

Because all tofu except the aseptically packaged silken is quite perishable, be sure to use it within two days of purchase. Once opened, store it in the refrigerator submerged in cold water in a covered container.

Simmered Succulent Tofu

SERVES 4

When squares of tofu are gently heated in dashi, they absorb the stock and become voluptuously succulent. The various garnishes provide all the necessary seasoning. Be sure to add the tofu to the dashi before heating the dashi, to prevent the tofu squares from overcooking and turning hard and crumbly. This warming dish is an ideal choice for a bitter cold night or a light winter lunch.

1 cup fresh-squeezed lemon (or lime) juice
1/2 cup reduced-sodium soy sauce
3 tablespoons mirin
1/2 cup small bonito flakes
4 shiso leaves, very thinly sliced
2 scallions, roots and top cut off, and thinly sliced
5 cups dashi
Two 1-pound blocks silken or cotton tofu

1. Blend the lemon juice, soy, and mirin in a small bowl to create a dipping sauce.
2. Place the bonito flakes in a small dish and the slivered shiso leaves and scallions on a small plate. Bring these garnishes to the table, along with 4 small bowls for the dipping sauce.
3. Place the dashi in a deep, 3-quart oven-to-table casserole. Although you will be cooking the tofu uncovered, the casserole should have a lid so that when you bring it to the table from the stove, you can cover it and keep the tofu hot. Gently rinse the tofu under cold water. Cut each block into large bite-size squares and add them to the dashi. Turn the heat to medium. The tofu cubes will swell and puff as the dashi heats. When the dashi is almost boiling, reduce the heat to low and gently simmer the tofu cubes for 4 minutes. When you remove the casserole from the flame, cover it and set it on a trivet in the center of the table.
4. To serve, let each diner pour approximately 2 tablespoons of dipping sauce into a small bowl. Using a small ladle, retrieve a few tofu cubes from the hot dashi, along with a little extra dashi, and add to the small bowl. Season the tofu with the garnishes as desired.

Tokyo Kitchen Tip

To avoid a spongy or undesirable texture and flavor, don't overcook the tofu.

WASABI

Wasabi is a popular Japanese condiment that suffuses the palate with a mixture of spice and heat. Unlike the horseradish plant, which grows in soil, wasabi grows in cold, shallow streams high in the mountains of Japan. The rhizome portion of the wasabi plant, which is the edible part, is about 1 inch in diameter and ranges from 3 to 6 inches long.

Wasabi is expensive to harvest and cultivate, which is why most stores sell a cheap substitute under the wasabi name. If you've ever eaten sushi or sashimi at a modestly priced Japanese restaurant, chances are you've been served a small cone of light green paste fabricated primarily from mustard and/or horseradish powder and green food coloring. It's acrid, fiery, and flavorless and bears little resemblance to freshly grated wasabi.

A good alternative to buying fresh wasabi and grating it right before you use it is pregrated real wasabi paste in a tube. At www.freshwasabi.com, you can order the tube, or you can even buy wasabi plants for your own cultivation if you're feeling really ambitious about having the genuine article.

Beyond its use in sushi and sashimi, wasabi often accompanies cold soba noodles, chilled tofu, and various fish and grilled chicken dishes.

YOUR TOKYO KITCHEN SHOPPING LIST:
WHERE TO SHOP
Look for At . . .

	Supermarket	Japanese or Asian Specialty Grocery Store	Online
Bonito (fish) flakes	X	X	X
Daikon (Japanese giant white radish)	X	X	
Japanese-style short-grain rice	X	X	X
Japanese teas	X	X	X
Mirin (cooking wine)	X	X	X
Miso (fermented soybean paste)*	X	X	X
Noodles: soba and udon	X	X	X
Oils: canola oil, sesame oil	X	X	X
Oil: rice bran oil		X	X
Rice Vinegar	X	X	X
Rice wine (sake)	Liquor Store		
Sea vegetables: hijiki, kombu, nori	X	X	X
Sesame seeds (goma)	X	X	X
Shiso		X	
Soy sauce (shoyu)*	X	X	X
Tofu	X	X	
Wasabi	X	X	X

* Look for low- or reduced-sodium soy sauce and miso.

JAPANESE HOME COOKING DEMYSTIFIED
Japanese Food Means . . .

THE MYTH	THE REALITY
Restaurant event	Home cooking too
Sushi only	Dozens of healthy, delicious dishes
Difficult to prepare	Easy and fun
Complex and inaccessible	Simple and attainable
Mysterious	Warm and familiar
Expensive	Surprisingly affordable
Every once in a while	Everyday lifestyle
Hard-to-find ingredients	Easy-to-find ingredients
Buying a lot of specialty cookware	Buying a couple of new items
Chopsticks required	Chopsticks strictly optional
Foreign	As American as apple pie and pizza!

CHAPTER 5

The Seven Pillars of
Japanese Home Cooking

If you have a pleasant experience eating something you have never tasted before, your life will be lengthened by seventy-five days.

Better than a feast elsewhere is a meal at home of tea and rice.

—Japanese folk sayings

THERE ARE SEVEN PILLARS of Japanese home cooking and they rest upon a culinary tradition that has endured for more than a thousand years.

It's true that in recent years these pillars—the fish, vegetables, rice, soy, noodles, tea, and fruit that have been relied upon by Japanese women and their families for generations—have been adapted and combined with Western food techniques and ingredients to create a multitude of new styles and dishes. But there has been a consistency to the basic outlines of most of these pillars that we can trace back not just to samurai times, but possibly even to the dawn of Japan's history—right back to the dinner table of the woman who may have created the Japanese nation itself.

Her name was Queen Himiko.

The little we know about her is based not on Japanese records (there weren't any yet) but on Chinese court histories. In the decades before the year A.D. 180, apparently, a series of male tribal leaders tried in vain to govern portions of the area now known as Japan, but succeeded only in presiding over conditions of full-blown chaos and constant warfare.

"Then a woman named Himiko appeared," according to the *Wei chi* chronicle, a historical account written by Chinese diplomats, "thereupon the people agreed upon a woman for their ruler." Himiko was a sorceress, or shaman, the chronicle reported, who "occupied herself with magic and sorcery, bewitching the people." Today we might call her a charismatic spiritual leader.

Whatever Himiko's leadership secret was, she seems to have made a blazing mark on history.

In A.D. 180, Queen Himiko united dozens of neighboring tribes into a single state called Wa, or Yamatai-koku, which set the stage for the emergence of the earliest Japanese nation-state. She surrounded herself with no fewer than one thousand female lieutenants and a SWAT team of armed bodyguards on hair-trigger alert, and installed them all in a heavily defended palace surrounded by towers and stockades. Reaching out to the neighboring kingdom, she exchanged diplomats with China and received boxfuls of exquisite gifts from the Chinese court, including a hundred bronze mirrors, which she may have used in shamanistic ceremonies and sun worship.

Her people prospered in peace as fisherman and farmers, eating a diet heavy in vegetables, rice, and fish. She herself was so finicky about her food that she selected one man to serve as her chef on an exclusive basis. He must have been quite a multitasker, as he also acted as her public spokesman and wardrobe director. Perhaps it was he who influenced the fashions of the time—women wearing stylish hood-robes over their intricately looped hair, men sporting headbands made of bark.

Queen Himiko ruled for at least sixty years.

By the time she died in 248, she was probably at least eighty years old—which is not too far from the current Japanese women's projected life expectancy of eighty-five years.

Queen Himiko's grand burial mound has never been found, nor has the location of her palace. But over the last century, archaeologists have been discovering bronze mirrors of Chinese design in different locations across Japan, many of them with dates and inscriptions corresponding with the Age of Himiko.

According to Japanese food scholar Hisao Nagayama, Queen Himiko's royal menu would have featured dishes like grilled river fish, scallions, rice, herbs, wild boar, chestnuts and walnuts, wakame seaweed, and mountain vegetables. On January 24, 2005, schoolchildren in the Japanese city of Joyo paid a special tribute to Queen Himiko, and to the traditional ways of eating, by re-creating what she would have eaten on a typical day on the throne. In honor of their long-ago queen, every schoolchild enjoyed a "Himiko lunch," which consisted of rice, clear soup with clams, and one of my favorite vegetable dishes—simmered country potatoes.

Together, let's now explore the seven pillars of Japanese home cooking, and how to make the dishes that incorporate them, including a miso soup with clams that is good enough to have appeared on the royal table at Queen Himiko's palace.

I am walking across the most famous bridge in Tokyo. No, actually I'm almost running, since I'm trying to catch up with my mother, who flies through the streets of Tokyo at lightning speed.

I don't know if it's her diet or her genes, but this woman can really move.

It's early morning and we're heading to one of her favorite culinary destinations, and one of the greatest spectacles in the city: the daily extravaganza of money, blood, and choreographed chaos known as the Tsukiji fish market.

This is the world olympics of fish.

The vast Tsukiji market is where the most elite of the ocean's creatures go to be paraded, poked, haggled over, butchered, and auctioned off to the highest bidder. Every day, a mind-numbing five million pounds of fish, living and dead, travels into this labyrinthine fifty-six-acre complex of warehouses, hangars, and loading docks, destined for the restaurants, department stores, bento boxes, and dinner plates of what may be the world's most fish-besotted people.

To get there, my mother and I have walked through the streets of downtown Tokyo, and the bridge we are now crossing, the Nihonbashi, or Japan Bridge, was once the starting point of the old trade routes to Kyoto and Osaka, the center of a merchant culture that rose up on the back of the almighty fish. Fashioned of wood in 1603 and rebuilt in stone in 1911, the dragon-studded Nihonbashi is one of the few vestigial echoes of an earlier age—the Edo era—that has survived until today, though it is nearly overwhelmed by the modern expressway that soars directly over our heads.

To get to the Tsukiji fish market, we are traveling into the lost, invisible heart of Edo (which was the name Tokyo had from 1603 to 1868). The memory of old Edo and Edo culture has a kind of poignancy for some Japanese, who continue to cherish a nearly forgotten vision of a distant past that can still be glimpsed—fleetingly—here and there. You can sense it in the shadows that line the twisting and narrow side streets, and see it in the tiny houses and proud mom-and-pop shops that specialize in items ranging from dried sea vegetables to Japanese confectionary. Many of these shops are run by families who can trace their lineage back to Edo times.

If you were to step through a time warp and walk these same streets in the early years of Edo—say, 1690 or so—and you peeked into a private home at dinnertime, you might spot a home-cooked meal almost identical to what my mother has planned for tonight: rice, miso soup, pickled vegetables, simmered vegetables, tofu, and a piece of grilled fish.

You'd also see streams of travelers swarming toward the Nihonbashi Bridge, heading out for the provinces—many of them salesmen bearing cartloads and basketfuls of preserved fish. And according to an eyewitness from the year 1692, many of them would be carrying printed food guides with them, listing the best places to eat along the road ahead, complete with prices. This was more than 200 years before the first Michelin guide appeared in France—and nearly 300 years before Zagat!

The fish market used to be located in the Nihonbashi district. In the early Edo period, the shogun (or military ruler) Ieyasu Tokugawa gave fishermen the right to operate in Edo Bay. They were to bring the freshest, best fish directly to him in Edo Castle. Any remaining fish could be sold to the local people in Nihonbashi—the beginnings of the vast market that eventually developed there.

The great earthquake of 1923 burned the original fish market to the ground, and the new market that was built is in the Tsukiji area, about 1½ miles southwest of Nihonbashi.

Walking through the narrow streets of the Kyobashi and Ginza neighborhoods, my mother and I eventually arrive at the Tsukiji market, near the convergence of the Sumida and Tsukiji rivers. We smell it even before we see it, intense aromas of the ocean announcing its presence.

If Japanese food has a Temple of Apollo, this is it.

We are approaching the First Pillar of Japanese home cooking, fish.

THE FIRST PILLAR: FISH

Stepping into the outer precincts of Tsukiji, we enter a ballet of scurrying workmen with handcarts and speeding forklifts bearing giant fish.

In the distance we can see monster ice machines disgorging waterfalls of ice into crates, water splashing everywhere, and salespeople dashing about in a frenzy of activity as curtains of mist rise from rows of slaughtered tuna.

Professional-looking guys with clipboards and badges march by, looking like traders on the floor of the New York Stock Exchange, except for their long rubber boots. In fact, this really is kind of a stock exchange, and the very valuable commodity being traded is fish. Every morning at five o'clock there is a boisterous national fish auction in the market's inner auditorium. Bids are screamed. Prices are argued. Japanese TV news reports on tuna price gyrations like a key economic index.

This market is geared for industrial-strength fish brokers and buyers, but civilian shoppers like us are allowed in too. I've been coming here with my mother ever since I was a little girl, because she likes to wheel and deal with the pros for the absolute freshest fish right off the boat or via air express delivery, from as near as the prefecture of Chiba across Tokyo Bay and as far away as South Africa, Chile, Maine, Scotland, and Norway.

At the end of every December we would come here to stock up on special New Year's dish ingredients like the gorgeous sea bream (whose Japanese name, *"tai,"* suggests "fortune"), shrimp, sashimi, caviar, clams, and assortments of seaweed. The highlight of these mornings for me was a late breakfast at one of the bustling world's-highest-class sushi restaurants on the edge of the market.

This is where food professionals go to eat when they've finished a day of fish deal making. The decor is stripped down and the food is cheap. But—what food! The sushi here not only melts in your mouth, it practically breaks your heart.

We turn a corner into Tsukiji's "outer market" and as far as the eye can see are aisles crammed with little specialty stalls and shops selling dried fish flakes, knives, sushi trays, ceramic plates, and exquisite kaiseki dish ingredients and seasonings.

Some of these family shops go back fifteen generations, back to when Greater Tokyo was not the confederation of smaller cities and wards totaling 30 million people that it is today, but barely a few hundred shacks surrounding a dilapidated castle. Every shop sign and interior in this part of the market has a patina of age, lending a real sense of history to the place.

We stop at a family-owned mushroom shop and buy eleven pounds of dried premium shiitake mushrooms for 3,500 yen ($32) from the proprietor, a woman my mother made fast friends with when they were both standing on line for tickets for a kabuki performance.

I wander off toward where the smells get stronger and the noises louder. And there it is: the vast frenzied interior market of the world's largest fish fair.

This is the Big Show.

A team of workmen is assaulting a 300-pound tuna with electric saws. Armadas of lobster drift nervously in plastic buckets. Crabs scamper and eels wriggle on piles of packed ice.

Every conceivable ocean resident is represented in this aquatic hall of fame: salmon, blowfish, barracuda, squid, octopus, shrimp, jellyfish, mackerel, and some sluggy, murky things with antennae and tentacles that look fresh from an *Aliens* casting call.

During the peak year-end shopping season, wrote anthropologist Theodore Bestor, "the inner market aisles are clogged with middle-aged housewives in expensive fur jackets and gold jewelry, well-dressed elderly men trailing a couple of grandchildren, and small clusters of women in their early twenties in fashionable ski parkas. Children—almost never seen in the inner market at other times in the year—are everywhere. Stall keepers watch with restrained displeasure as small children occasionally poke fingers into the strange fish, but they tend to hold their tongues; the culprits might turn out to be the beloved grandchildren of a prized customer."

———

There's no question about it—Japan is a fish-crazed nation.

Fish is the meat of Japan. Japanese people eat fish for breakfast, lunch, and dinner. They snack on rice balls sprinkled with fish. They eat raw tuna, trout sushi, teriyaki cod, miso-simmered mackerel, clam soup, fried scallops, shrimp tempura, rice vinegar-marinated octopus, and grilled squid.

And in this nation of hard-core fish fans, one fish is king: salmon. It is even more coveted than tuna, which is a very close contender. Every fall and winter, uncounted multitudes of salmon surge into the northern rivers and streams of Japan in search of romance amid the pebbles of a cool riverbed, and every spring their love children flock out into the Pacific Ocean, on voyages that often culminate on the business end of a Japanese chopping knife.

Japanese love the taste of salmon,* and they've found endless ways to enjoy it. There's salmon steak, vinegared salmon skin, salmon roe seasoned with soy sauce over rice (*ikura-donburi*), and salt-cured salmon kidney (*mefun*). In the north, in snowy Hokkaido, salmon is the star of one-pot hot casserole dishes like Ishikari-nabe and akiaji-nabe. In ancient Japan, salted and preserved salmon was carried from across the country to the capital as tax payments, and as gifts to the imperial household.

Japan's fish craze has roots in the seventh century A.D., when an especially devout Buddhist emperor issued a sweeping animal rights decree outlawing the eating of all land animals. The royal edict was in force for twelve hundred years, until 1873, leaving untold millions of cows, pigs, and chickens to frolic happily in the fields more or less unmolested (although there were always closet Japanese meat lovers who managed to

---

* Or sake, as the locals call it, not to be confused with the rice wine that happens to have the same spelling.

sneak the occasional piece of bootleg cooked chicken or barbe-cued horse nugget).

This edict was great news for cows, and bad news for fish. With a shortage of wide-open range space, cows were never that common in Japan to begin with, so production of butter, cream, and cheese never really took off either, not until fairly recently. Even today, although Japanese have certainly been given the message that milk is good for you, they drink less than a third of the amount of milk per person compared with the United States, the United Kingdom, France, and Germany.

Conversely, Japan consumes nearly 10 percent of the world's fish, although it makes up only about 2 percent of the world's population. Japanese people eat 150 pounds of fish per person each year, over four times the world average of 35 pounds. The ancient habits die hard—fortunately for the health of this na-tion of fish eaters.

According to the experts, all this fish may be a key factor in Japan's number one ranking in the world in both overall longevity and in healthy longevity. "Dozens of studies have found that eating fish lowers your risk of having a heart attack or stroke," reported the *Harvard Health Letter* in 2003. "Fish consumption has long been recognized as important in the prevention of CAD (coronary artery disease). Protective effects are most likely related to the cardiovascular benefits of omega-3 fatty acids."

Eating all that fish means that the Japanese are swimming (culinarily speaking) in a rich ocean of polyunsaturated omega-3 fatty acids, which are found in particularly high quantities in fish like salmon, mackerel, sardines, and trout. Since heart disease is the biggest killer in the developed world, the fact that omega-3s have been linked to cardiovascular health is seen by experts as a major clue for understanding Japanese longevity.

Dr. Michel de Lorgeril, chief scientist investigator for the French National Center for Scientific Research, and one of the top research experts on the French and Mediterranean diets, is one of those who make that connection. In considering why Japan has both high longevity and low cardiac mortality, he tells us, "My feeling is that the traditional Japanese diet is very important." Dr. de Lorgeril observes that, compared with the Japanese diet, Western diets "are severely deficient in omega-3 fatty acids."

A growing body of research points to the advantages of a diet rich in omega-3s. In a paper published in 2005, Dr. Mark Moyad of the University of Michigan Medical Center wrote, "One of the most intriguing current and future impacts on public health may come from a greater intake of omega-3 fatty acids," particularly EPA and DHA, two of the three omega-3s. "The omega-3 fatty acids continue to accumulate research that suggests they may prevent a variety of diverse chronic diseases and potentially some acute clinical scenarios."

"If you really want to do something heart healthy for yourself," declared cardiologist Dr. Robert A. Vogel of the University of Maryland School of Medicine at a 2002 conference sponsored by the American College of Cardiology, "either eat a little fish every day or take a gram or two of dietary fatty-acid-rich fish oil capsules."

The benefits may not be limited just to heart disease. Dr. Rudolph Tanzi, a professor at Harvard Medical School and the director of genetics and aging research at Massachusetts General

Hospital, reports that "omega-3 fatty acids from fish are protective for Alzheimer's, cardiovascular disease, rheumatoid arthritis, and several forms of cancer."

Another authority who sings the praises of omega-3s is Philip C. Calder, professor of nutritional immunology at Britain's University of Southampton School of Medicine. He has been studying the health effects of omega-3s for nearly a decade. "I have no doubt that fish consumption is a key player in the better health in Japan," Professor Calder reports, "mainly because of the consumption of long chain omega-3 fatty acids found in fish." Research in Europe and North America, he says, offer "good evidence that fish and omega-3 fatty acids protect against cardiovascular disease and it seems likely that they protect against some other disorders too, such as some cancers." He adds, "Fish also contain important minerals like selenium and iodine and certain antioxidants. These are likely protective against cardiovascular and malignant diseases, and inflammatory conditions."

Professor Calder boils down the lessons of the traditional Japanese diet to two words: "Eat fish!" The American Heart Association agrees, recommending that adults eat fish, particularly fatty fish, at least twice a week. So do the federal government's nutrition guidelines issued in early 2005, which recommend: "Choose fish more often for lunch or dinner. Look for fish rich in omega-3 fatty acids, such as salmon, trout, and herring." The Food and Drug Administration has approved use of a qualified health claim for products containing fish oils, stating, "Supportive but not conclusive research shows that consumption of EPA and DHA omega-3 fatty acids may reduce the risk of coronary heart disease."

Experts around the world are examining the possible positive impact of omega-3s not only on physiological conditions but on psychosocial conditions as well, including depression, aggression, suicide, hostility, personality disorder, and even homicide rates.

———

But wait—there's a major "catch" in this fishy paradise. Some fish stand accused of being contaminated. And some of these fish are guilty as charged.

For example, according to the Environmental Defense Fund's Oceans Alive project, several types of fish have been the subject of health advisories for mercury, PCBs, dioxin, or pesticides—including shark, swordfish, tilefish, grouper, wild sturgeon, bluefin tuna, and, I am sad to report, a type of salmon that happens to be very common in North American supermarkets: Atlantic salmon. Even the friendly, delicious workhorse albacore tuna gets a consumption warning due to mercury, dioxin, and PCBs.

Over the last two years, the Food and Drug Administration and the Environmental Protection Agency have advised pregnant women and women who may become pregnant, as well as nursing mothers and young children, not to eat shark, swordfish, king mackerel, or tilefish due to pollutants. Both agencies recommend that people not eat the same kind of fish more than once a week, to protect against excessive intake of mercury.

But here's the good news: this still leaves many types of fish that the Oceans Alive Web site classifies as both free of contamination warnings *and* farmed in an ecologically sound manner. This "eco best" list includes farmed striped bass, northern shrimp from the North Atlantic, snow crab from Canada, Florida stone crab, farmed sturgeon, Atlantic herring, black cod from Alaska (or sablefish), and several fish that are especially rich in omega-3 fatty acids: Atlantic mackerel, sardines, and farmed oysters.

For a salmon lover like myself, the great news is that all wild salmon from Alaska, including chinook, coho, pink, and sockeye, whether fresh, frozen, or canned, makes the eco-best cut. Moreover, these varieties of salmon all boast more than 1 gram of omega-3s per 100 gram serving. And again, it doesn't matter whether the salmon is fresh, frozen, or canned. According to the Center for Science in the Public Interest, canned salmon has the same amount of omega-3s per serving as fresh or frozen. More good news: none of these types of salmon is currently the subject of any consumption advisories.

No matter how you slice it, Alaska salmon rules!

———

Fish can be a great way to get omega-3s, but the flip side of Japan's fish craze reveals another possible health clue: the high Japanese fish consumption means less consumption of red meat, which is high in the saturated fats implicated in cardiovascular disease. According to the latest estimates of *The Economist* magazine's Intelligence Unit, Japanese currently eat 100 pounds of meat per person per year. The corresponding annual figures are 285 pounds in the United States annually, 225 pounds in France, and 180 pounds in Great Britain and Germany.

Personally, I love fish not only for its health benefits but even more so for its flavors and the many different ways we can cook it.

The tangy ocean flavor of littleneck, Manila, or New Zealand clams in a clear soup is distinct and unforgettable. Fish with meaty white flesh like Pacific halibut are great for teriyaki dishes. When the fish cooks, the flesh is transformed into shimmering white flakes of meat that seem to yearn to be smothered in teriyaki sauce.

Some fish simply dissolve in your mouth, like sole or amberjack. I always enjoy a dish of grilled Atlantic mackerel garnished with a small mound of grated daikon and a few drops of soy sauce. Another of my favorites is sardines simmered in ginger–soy sauce broth.

I love salmon for its rich, meaty taste and the multitude of ways it can be prepared: simply grilled, as a filling for rice balls, over rice with salmon caviar, smoked and rolled with spicy daikon sprouts—and those are only a few of its myriad uses.

Just thinking about all these fish, I am getting hungry for a bowl of miso soup with clams.

———

Miso Soup with Short-Neck Clams

SERVES 4

I love how the briny flavor of the clams combines with the earthy-tasting miso. They add an appealing punch to this traditional Japanese soup.

12 short-neck (also called littleneck) clams in the shell
  (about ³/₄ pound)

¹/₄ cup fine-ground sea salt

9 cups cold water

1 tablespoon sake

2¹/₂ tablespoons red or white miso (or use a combination of both)

2 scallions, roots and rough portion of the tops cut off,
  and thinly sliced

1. Scrub the clams under cold water to eliminate any dirt from the
   shells, then rinse the clams in several changes of water until the
   water runs clear. To eliminate any grit inside the shells, dissolve
   the salt in 4 cups of the cold water and soak the clams in the salt
   solution in the refrigerator for 20 minutes. Drain and then rinse.
2. Place the remaining 5 cups of cold water in a large saucepan.
   Add the clams. Bring the liquid to a boil, then add the sake.
   Skim foam from the surface of the liquid with a ladle. As soon
   as the clams open, which should be only a few minutes after
   the water comes to a boil, they are cooked. Turn the heat to
   low and transfer 1 cup of stock from the saucepan to a medium bowl. Whisk in the miso until it dissolves. Turn off the
   heat and pour the miso mixture back into the hot broth and
   gently stir (to avoid knocking the clams out of their shells).
3. Lay out 4 small soup bowls. Using kitchen tongs, arrange 3
   clams in each bowl. Ladle the soup over the clams and garnish
   with scallions. Place a bowl in the center of the table to hold the
   discarded shells.

Tokyo Kitchen Tips

You do not need to use dashi for this soup because the clams season the cooking liquid with their own rich taste.

It's important to cook the clams only until they have just opened; otherwise, they will become tough.

———

Smoked Salmon Rolls with Shiso and Kaiware

SERVES 4

These succulent salmon bundles make a wonderful East-meets-West sort of nibble to serve with drinks. You can make them earlier in the day, seal the platter with plastic wrap, and refrigerate them until ready to serve. Because the rind and pith of a lemon can be quite bitter (and not to everyone's taste), try to find very thin-skinned lemons to use in this appetizer. Alternatively, omit the lemon slice from the salmon bundles and serve them with lemon wedges, letting guests squeeze a bit of lemon juice over their salmon bundles before eating them. Kaiware are daikon sprouts with tender white stems and round green leaves. They are mildly spicy, so they make a great garnish. You can often find them in the sprout section of stores that carry a variety of sprouts.

> One 2½- to 3-ounce package fresh kaiware (daikon sprouts)
> 12 slices thinly sliced smoked salmon (about 8 ounces)
> 5 shiso leaves, cut into very thin ribbons

12 paper-thin half-moon slices of a very thin-skinned
lemon (or 1 lemon cut into 4 wedges)

1. Slice off the spongy white portion of the kaiware. Divide the sprouts into 12 little bundles.

2. For each salmon roll, lay a slice of smoked salmon on a clean work surface with the long portion running vertically down the work surface (like a necktie). Place a pinch of slivered shiso toward the bottom portion of the salmon slice. Lay a portion of the kaiware over the shiso with the little green leaves of the sprouts sticking out slightly toward the right so they will peek out of the salmon roll when you roll it up. Place a lemon slice, if using, over the sprout stems. Working from bottom to top, roll the salmon upward to create a neat bundle. Continue making the salmon rolls in this manner until you have used up all your ingredients. You will have 12 rolls.

3. Arrange the rolls on a serving plate (with lemon wedges if not using the lemon slices).

Salmon-Edamame Burger

SERVES 4

Bright green edamame pumps up the protein in these juicy salmon burgers. You can buy frozen, blanched, shelled edamame at select stores, including Whole Foods. Panko, Japanese bread crumbs, is a modern ingredient, which makes a light, crunchy crust. (The term is a fusion of the French word for bread, "pain," with "ko," which means "powder" in Japanese.) Unlike the bread crumbs you are probably used to, panko have a texture that is more like flakes than crumbs. You can find panko in the Asian food section of supermarkets, as well as in gourmet food stores and Japanese grocery stores.

Enjoy these fish patties drizzled with a little soy and grated daikon.

> One 1-inch-long chunk fresh peeled gingerroot
> 1 cup blanched shelled edamame (thawed, if frozen)
> 1 pound skinless, boneless salmon fillet, cut into small
>   chunks
> ½ cup finely chopped onion
> ½ cup finely chopped green bell pepper
> 1 tablespoon sake
> 1½ teaspoons reduced-sodium soy sauce
> ¼ teaspoon salt
> Freshly ground black pepper
> ½ cup all-purpose flour
> 1 cup panko
> 1 large egg
> 4 cups of canola oil or rice bran oil
> 4 small sprigs mitsuba or Italian parsley

1. Place the chunk of gingerroot in a food processor fitted with a metal blade and process until minced, scraping down the sides of the work bowl one or two times, as necessary. Add the shelled edamame and pulse until minced. Transfer the mixture to a large bowl.
2. Place the raw salmon chunks in the food processor and process until ground. Transfer to the bowl with the edamame mixture,

and add the onion, green pepper, sake, soy, salt, and several grinds of black pepper. Stir the mixture until well blended.

3. Lightly wet your hands. Form the salmon mixture into 8 patties and set them aside.

4. Put flour on one large plate and panko on another. Beat the egg in a shallow, medium-size bowl. One by one, coat each salmon patty in the flour, then in the beaten egg, and finally in the panko. Gently remove the patty from the panko and press it between your hands.

5. Heat the oil in a large deep skillet and bring it to 340°F. If you don't have a thermometer, test the oil with a panko flake. If the panko flake rises and immediately turns golden, then the oil is hot enough. Gently lower the salmon patties into the oil, and fry for 2 minutes on each side, or until nicely golden brown. Remove the patties from the oil and place on a metal rack to drain excess oil.

6. To serve, lay out 4 plates and arrange 2 patties on each plate. Garnish with the mitsuba (or the Italian parsley).

Shrimp and Vegetable Tempura

SERVES 4

Although I grew up eating tempura and it is one of my favorite dishes, to be honest, I was afraid of making it. My mother cooks it beautifully, and without any apparent effort. But to me, tempura seemed to present so many challenges—like deep-frying it at the right temperature, making the batter light and crisp, and serving it while it's still hot—that I was daunted. When my mom took me through the process step by step, I discovered it actually wasn't that difficult—and the taste is so good that I have real trouble finding the words to describe it.

> 1 cup dashi (page 52)
> ¼ cup reduced-sodium soy sauce
> ¼ cup mirin
> ½ pound Japanese eggplant (about 2 medium egg-plants)
> 1 small sweet potato or jewel yam, washed, stems cut off, and unpeeled
> 1 small white potato, washed
> 1 medium onion, trimmed and peeled
> ¼ small acorn squash, washed, stems cut off, and seeds removed
> 1 green bell pepper
> 4 shiitake mushrooms, stems trimmed
> 12 large shrimp
> About 5 cups canola oil or rice bran oil, for deep-frying
> 1 large egg
> ½ cup ice water
> 1 cup all-purpose flour
> ½ cup of finely grated daikon, drained

1. To prepare the dipping sauce, combine the dashi, soy, and mirin in a medium saucepan. Bring to a boil, and then remove from heat. Set aside and let cool to room temperature.
2. Prepare the vegetables. Cut off the stem cap of each eggplant,

and cut each eggplant into ½-inch-thick rounds. Slice both potatoes into ¼-inch-thick rounds. Cut the onion into 12 wedges. Cut the squash quarter into ¼-inch-thick wedges. Core the pepper and cut in half; remove the seeds and cut each half into 3 long slices. Use the mushrooms whole.

3. Devein each shrimp, and peel the shell, except the last shell segment closest to the tail and the tail itself.

4. Prepare the deep fryer by filling a wok or large deep skillet with enough oil so it is at least 3 inches deep (about 5 cups). Heat the oil over medium heat until it reaches 350°F. If you don't have a thermometer, test the oil with a tiny square of fresh bread. If the bread rises and immediately turns golden, then the oil is hot enough.

5. Just before frying, make the tempura batter. (Making it too much in advance will cause it to become gluey.) In a medium bowl, whisk the egg with the ice water. Then add all the flour at once and with a fork or chopsticks mix ever so slightly, so that there are still lumps of flour floating on the surface of the bat-ter. This will keep the batter light.

6. To fry the vegetables, dip pieces into the batter, shake off the excess, and add to the hot oil. Add only five or six items to the oil at one time to keep the oil from cooling, and gently swish them around to prevent the oil from getting too hot and smoking. Fry each item until golden and cooked through; then remove it from the oil with a mesh scoop (or slotted spoon) and drain on a metal rack lined with paper towels. Let the oil return to 350°F between each batch of frying. Most vegetables will need 3 to 5 minutes of frying until tender and cooked through, but exact timing will vary, depending upon the hardness of the vegetables. Test for doneness by piercing the vegetable with a wooden skewer. You

should be able to slide it easily all the way through. Cook the shrimp last. They will cook in about 40 seconds.

7. To serve, line 4 individual serving plates with absorbent paper. Arrange a portion of vegetables and shrimp on each and bring to the table. Place the grated daikon on another plate and pour approximately ⅓ cup of sauce per person into a small bowl. Let diners season their dipping sauce with as much grated daikon as desired. Replenish the sauce and daikon as needed.

Teriyaki Fish

SERVES 4

Here's a homemade version of a Japanese classic. Fresh teriyaki sauce is so simple to make that you might never want to buy the bottled version again.

> Four 4-ounce fish fillets (each ½-inch thick) of wild Alaska
> salmon, farmed striped bass, or Pacific halibut
> 1 tablespoon canola oil or rice bran oil

Marinade

2 tablespoons sake
4 teaspoons reduced-sodium soy sauce

Teriyaki Sauce

¼ cup mirin

2 tablespoons reduced-sodium soy sauce

1 teaspoon granulated sugar

1. Make the marinade by blending the sake and soy sauce in a shallow dish. Place the fish fillets flesh side down in the dish (if using a fish with skin, such as salmon), and marinate for 10 minutes.

2. Make the teriyaki sauce by blending together the mirin, soy sauce, and sugar in a small bowl. Whisk the mixture together until the sugar has dissolved.

3. Heat the oil in large skillet over medium-high heat. Using a paper towel, gently blot each fish fillet on both sides to absorb any excess marinade. Place the fillets in the skillet (skin side down, if the fish has skin) and cook for 5 minutes. Turn the fillets and cook for 1 minute more.

4. Transfer the fish to a large plate (the fish will finish cooking in the teriyaki sauce) and peel off any skin.

5. With a paper towel, wipe out any excess grease from the skillet. Place the skillet back over medium-high heat and add the teriyaki sauce. Bring to a boil, reduce the heat to medium, and simmer the sauce for 1 minute. Add the fish. Tip the pan slightly and spoon some of the teriyaki sauce over the fillets. Cook them for 1 minute, or until the center portion is just cooked through.

6. Arrange the fish on individual serving plates and top with the hot teriyaki sauce.

THE SECOND PILLAR: VEGETABLES

As my mother and I emerge from the Tsukiji fish market and walk through the densely packed Tokyo side streets, I am reminded of a man singing a song from long ago.

He was singing about the second pillar of Japanese home cooking—vegetables.

I grew up in a vegetable-rich world.

One of my most vivid childhood memories was of hearing the "sweet potato man" pulling a two-wheel wagon with cooking gear through the backstreets of Japan in wintertime, singing his chant, "Yaki-imo, ishi-yaki-imo!" This basically means "Come and get my succulent stone-grilled sweet potatoes!"

In the United States, you have the ice cream truck and its signature melody, which gathers all the children within earshot. Our version was a wagon, and the treat we flocked to was a vegetable that was sold by the pound. The sweet potato man walked from street to street, singing his sweet potato song, the wheels of his wagon sending the fallen leaves flying through the air. He would often arrive in our neighborhood in midafternoon, when my sister and I were home from school.

As soon as we heard the sweet potato song, we would beg our mother for some small change, then dash into the street to chase down the vendor. I'd ask for four medium-size sweet potatoes for the family—one for each of us. Wearing a pair of cotton work gloves to keep his fingers from being burned, he'd grab some shapely sweet potatoes from his mobile grill, weigh them on the measuring scale attached to his wagon, wrap them up in a newspaper, and hand them to me. I can still smell their rich aroma and picture their scorched burgundy skin.

Sweet potato men still travel through the backstreets of Japan during the winter, only now they travel in minivans, not on foot.

The tradition of mobile food carts in Tokyo dates back to the 1780s, when a person walking down a busy street could expect to see a long line of carts parked along the side of the road and hear a cacophony of overlapping "sales songs" being sung simultaneously—a different song each for sushi, tempura, grilled eel, dumplings, dried squid, rice cakes, and steamed rice.

Today, as my mother and I closely inspect fresh produce at the Mitsukoshi department store, deciding what to buy for dinner, we are greeted by a different kind of music—the sounds of dozens of competing sales ladies singing welcomes over their little mountains of exquisite vegetables.

In Japan, people eat a wide range of mountain, root, field, and sea vegetables, some that are indigenous to Japan and many others that have been imported from overseas. Vegetables are often the lead player in a Japanese meal, and when Japanese mothers were asked in a poll to rank the home-cooked meals they most love to make for their families, "mixed vegetables simmered in seasoned broth" was the hands-down winner. Vegetables are also, of course, in many side dishes.

One vegetable even makes an appearance, to the surprise of the uninitiated, in Japanese desserts. Traditional Japanese sweets, known as wagashi, feature beans—most commonly, adzuki (small red beans), or else kidney beans, green beans, or soybeans. Wagashi come in many variations. There are mochi dumplings in a sweet red bean soup (*shiratama zenzai*), baked wheat flour buns with bean paste filling (*azuki manju*), adzuki bean filling sandwiched between two rice cracker wafers (*monaka*), and one of Japan's favorite sweets, a dense jellied treat made from bean paste called yokan. One product, green tea daifuku, manages to squeeze three of the country's favorite foods into one mouthful: green tea, soy powder, and bean paste, wrapped in sticky rice.

———

I am simply not rational on the subject of vegetables—not because I'm a health nut, but because they taste so good.

I think vegetables can be scandalously scrumptious. Give me a steaming dish of fresh, kaleidoscopically colorful veggies diced and stir-fried lovingly in a tiny bit of canola oil—vegetables like red bell pepper, green beans, yellow zucchini, purple eggplant, white onion, Tokyo negi, and cilantro, plus a bowl of cooked rice—and I am completely satisfied.

I cannot get enough of shiitake mushrooms. When simmered whole in a seasoned broth, they absorb the broth beautifully, and a bite into a meaty mushroom floods the mouth with a little burst of intense flavor. Sliced thinly, shiitake lends an elegant touch to a clear soup.

The creamy yellow flesh of eggplant becomes meltingly tender and almost sweet when it's grilled, broiled, or pan-fried and then garnished with a tiny bit of freshly grated gingerroot and soy sauce.

And then there are Japanese herbs: shiso, mitsuba, and myoga, to name a few. Shiso has a rich minty fragrance. Every time I open a package of shiso, I bury my nose in the leaves and inhale deeply. I use whole leaves of it to wrap my rice balls, and I often toss shredded shiso into my salads. In fact, I like shiso so much that I grow it in a planter at home.

Mitsuba, also known as trefoil or Japanese parsley, is a pretty garnish. I have included it in several of the recipes in this book, though Italian parsley is fine to use in its place. A sprig of mitsuba, knotted and set afloat in clear soup, is exquisite. Mitsuba also adds a nice touch on top of a salmon edamame burger.

Myoga is a relative of ginger, but it looks more like a narrow shallot. The top portion is reddish purple and it gradually fades to white toward the bottom. Thinly shredded, this fragrant herb garnishes blocks of chilled silken tofu, along with thinly sliced scallions. Sliced myoga adds a wickedly tasty touch to miso soup.

I enjoy vegetables so much that I constantly violate one of the cardinal rules of Western food behavior: I eat vegetables for breakfast. And I don't mean just potatoes—I mean all vegetables. At some point in time, it seems, someone issued an edict in certain sections of the world forbidding the use of vegetables at the breakfast table. I cannot obey.

In my mother's Tokyo kitchen, vegetables for breakfast are perfectly normal. My mother often makes vegetable egg soup for breakfast. The dish is light, filling, and flavorful. Even when she makes a Western-style breakfast with toasted bread, eggs, and coffee, she is sure to include a plate of salad.

Japanese moms consider the various types of seaweed, or sea vegetables, to be stars of the vegetable kingdom because of their nutritional value, often reminding their children to "eat your sea vegetables." Indeed, various forms of seaweed are good sources of vitamin C, fiber, potassium, and iodine.

Hiroko Mogi, a mother of four in her forties who lives in the city of Kawasaki, is a typical Japanese mom, in that she uses seaweed as a key ingredient in her home cooking every day. Her favorites are shredded black hijiki simmered in broth and wakame leaves in miso soup. "If you want to say it looks yucky, you may be right," she admits. But "if you taste it," she declares, "it's delicious."

I totally agree. I'm crazy about sea vegetables too—every bit as much as Western-style greens. There is a long tradition of love for those treasures from the sea. Over eleven centuries ago, the great Japanese writer Lady Murasaki rhapsodized about them in her tenth-century epic *The Tale of Genji:* "Rich seaweed tresses of the unplumbed ocean depths, a thousand fathoms long, you are mine and mine alone to watch daily as you grow."

I'm always looking for more ways to eat sea vegetables like kombu, nori, and wakame. I love thinly sliced cucumbers and wakame soaked in a rice vinegar dressing. Wakame is also delicious in a miso soup, with small blocks of silken tofu floating alongside it. I enjoy kombu in many forms, not just as a key component of dashi cooking stock. I use knotted strips of hydrated kombu as an ingredient for a one-pot dish called oden, which is cooked with blocks of daikon, fish cakes, and eggs. I also sprinkle a small quantity of simmered kombu on hot rice, and I pour green tea over rice and simmered kombu strips for a satisfying snack.

Nori seaweed is used to wrap many things in Japan: sushi rolls, rice balls, mochi cakes, rice crackers, and even strips of cheese. I shred sheets of nori and sprinkle them on rice, noodles, fish, and salad. My husband sprinkles them in his miso soup and on stir-fried vegetables. He also eats sweetly seasoned nori as it is, as a snack. Billy and I love shrimp, fish, and potatoes wrapped in nori, and then fried. Fried nori is crisp, adds an earthy snappy flavor, and goes well with many foods.

Your average Japanese woman is something of a vegetable connoisseur, with strong points of view on onions, eggplants, carrots, tomatoes, green peppers, lettuce, spinach, bamboo shoots, beets, yams, lotus root, and turnips; and with well-developed theories on the proper crispness of daikon, and on the best methods of cooking spinach or simmering gobo, which is a woodsy-tasting root vegetable otherwise known as burdock.

The vegetable aisle of a Tokyo supermarket looks a lot like yours. You'll find all of the vegetables just mentioned, as well as celery, cauliflower, peas, brussels sprouts, potatoes, cabbage, cucumber, mushrooms, beans, pumpkin, leafy greens, and scallions—and others I've probably forgotten to mention. You'll also see one of Japan's favorite veggies, the daikon, or giant white radish.

For land-based vegetables to be cooked at home, the one rule on which almost all Japanese women agree is that they must be fresh. The entire vegetable industry in Japan is geared to satisfying this nonnegotiable demand.

How do all these vegetables help Japanese people stay healthy?

Vegetables are hailed as superstars by nutritionists for many reasons. For one thing, vegetables are high-fiber, high-water complex carbohydrates, which help keep people's weight under control. Obesity expert Professor Kerin O'Dea explains that a key benefit of the vegetable-rich Japanese cuisine "is its bulk, or low energy density—meaning it will protect against overconsumption." And Professor Philip Calder, of Britain's University of Southampton, asserts that Japan's lower rates of obesity may relate in part to Japan's "better balance of carbohydrates: more complex carbohydrates, fewer simple."

What's great about vegetables, aside from their role in preventing obesity, is that they come fully equipped with vitamins. Minerals. Phytochemicals. Low calories. Low fat. High fiber. You name it. And then there are the antioxidants.

According to Professor Jerry W. Shay, chairman of geriatric research at the University of Texas Southwestern Medical Center, another reason the vegetable-rich traditional Japanese diet is a healthy one is that "vegetables contain potent antioxidants and these may help protect against cellular damage."

In their 2001 book *The Okinawa Program,* which was based on a twenty-five-year longevity study of people on the Japanese island of Okinawa, Bradley J. Willcox, D. Craig Willcox, and Makoto Suzuki wrote: "Never in the history of nutrition research has the evidence been more clear and consistent: a high-carbohydrate, low-calorie, plant-based diet is the best for long-term health. There is no doubt about it anymore, despite what you might have read in books advocating low-carb-high-protein diets. A well-balanced high-carbohydrate-low-calorie diet helps you stay slim, look youthful, and minimize your risk for heart disease, stroke, and cancer."

In the January 2004 issue of the *Mayo Clinic Proceedings,* cardiologist James H. O'Keefe Jr. and Professor Loren Cordain of Colorado State University wrote, "The one variable on which nearly all nutritional experts can agree is the need for increased intake of fruits and vegetables in our modern diet." Their advice was clear: "Consume these foods regularly in their natural and unprocessed state."

Some experts would like to see meat disappear from the diet altogether. "To increase the health of humans and the Earth that harbors us," says Dr. Rudolph Tanzi of Boston's Massachusetts General Hospital, "a vegetarian diet, or at least one devoid of all meats, is preferable. Clearly, the Japanese come closer to this goal on a day-to-day basis than Americans and Europeans."

For all the vegetables Japanese eat, some experts think they should eat even more, especially the fresh kind. Unfortunately, many of the vegetables consumed in Japan are pickled and salted, which contributes to what experts call an excessive amount of salt in the diet (implicated in the high rate of stomach cancer in Japan) and doesn't take full advantage of the nutrients available in fresh vegetables.

A Zen Approach to Food

The purest form of Japanese cooking is a rare, 100 percent vegetarian style called shojin ryori, or temple cuisine, which has been practiced by the Zen Buddhist clergy in Japan for more than eight hundred years. *"Shojin"* means "perseverance and devotion," and *"ryori"* means "cooking," or "cuisine." The theory behind shojin ryori is that food should enhance spiritual growth. Nothing is wasted. Only small portions of the simplest plant-based foods are used, but the result can be quite delicious.

A typical shojin meal might include stewed daikon with ground leek and miso sauce; steamed noodles topped with tofu paste, yam, and chopped wild chervil; and boiled spinach and steamed apple dressed with ground black sesame seeds.

There are five foundations of spirituality in Buddhism, and shojin cooking reflects the significance of the number five: it has five methods (raw, steamed, grilled, boiled, and fried), five colors (green, yellow, red, white, and black/purple) and five tastes (sweet, hot, bitter, sour, salty), and sometimes a sixth (*umami*, or savory).

My favorite aspect of shojin ryori is the five reflections, which are spoken by temple members prior to eating the meal.

THE FIVE ZEN FOOD REFLECTIONS

1. I reflect on the work that brings this food before me; let me see whence this food comes.

2. I reflect on my imperfections, on whether I am deserving of this offering of food.

3. Let me hold my mind free from preferences and greed.

4. I take this food as an effective medicine to keep my body in good health.

5. I accept this food so that I will fulfill my task of enlightenment.

Spinach with Sesame Seeds

SERVES 4

The ground sesame dressing used in this recipe has a rich roasted
nutty flavor and a hint of sweetness that really enhances the min-
erally saltiness of the spinach. It's a winning combination—so winning that once, when I brought this dish to a party, a chef friend of
mine kept it in her lap the entire night! The dressing also pairs
beautifully with cooked string beans, asparagus, and broccoli flo-
rets.

> One 1-pound bunch of spinach, roots and coarse bot-
>   tom of stems removed
> 2 1/2 tablespoons toasted and ground white sesame
>   seeds (page 111)
> 1 1/2 teaspoons granulated sugar
> 1 1/2 teaspoons reduced-sodium soy sauce
> Pinch of salt

1. Place the spinach in a large bowl filled with water and swish the
   leaves around to rinse off any dirt. If still gritty, lift the spinach
   out of the water, empty and refill the bowl, and repeat the
   process.
2. Bring a large saucepan of water to a boil. Turn down to medium-
   high heat, add the spinach and cook for 30 seconds, or until
   just wilted and still bright green. Drain and refresh under cold

water. Gently squeeze the spinach to release excess water.

3. Combine the toasted and ground sesame seeds in a small bowl with the sugar, soy, and a pinch of salt. Stir until well mixed.

4. Cut the spinach into 1-inch pieces, squeeze out excess water, and place in a small bowl. Pour the sesame mixture over the spinach and toss well to combine.

———

Stir-Fried Vegetables

SERVES 4

Japanese stir-fries focus on the pure natural taste of the vegetables and therefore tend to be seasoned more lightly than stir-fries from other parts of Asia. Enjoy this colorful mix with hot cooked brown rice for a healthy, fiber-rich meal. If you want to make it strictly vegetarian, you can omit the dashi and use the mushroom soaking water instead.

8 ounces extra firm tofu

8 dried shiitake mushrooms

1/4 cup dashi (page 52)

2 tablespoons reduced-sodium soy sauce

2 tablespoons sake

1/2 teaspoon salt

Freshly ground black pepper

2 tablespoons canola oil or rice bran oil

1 medium yellow onion, peeled, halved, and cut into thin crescents

2 medium carrots, trimmed, peeled, and diagonally cut
 into thin slices

1 medium Yukon gold potato (about 1/2 pound), diagonally halved, each half cut into 1/4-inch-thick slices

1/2 pound string beans, trimmed and diagonally cut in half

1 yellow summer squash, trimmed and diagonally
 halved, each half diagonally thinly sliced

1 red bell pepper, cored, seeded, and cut into thin strips

1. Rinse the tofu under cold water. Drain and cut into small dice.

2. Place the shiitake mushrooms in a small bowl and add 2 cups of
 water. Let soak for 20 minutes. Remove 1/4 cup of the mushroom
 soaking water (or 1/2 cup if making a vegetarian version) and
 place in a small bowl. Blend in the dashi (omit if making the
 vegetarian version), 1 tablespoon of the soy, the sake, and the salt.
 Add several grinds of pepper to this seasoning mixture.

3. Drain the mushrooms, squeeze gently to remove excess water.
 Cut off the stems. Cut each cap into thin slices.

4. Heat the oil in a wok or large sauté pan over medium-high
 heat. Add the onion and shiitake caps and stir-fry for 3 minutes.
 Add the carrots and potato slices and stir-fry for 3 minutes. Stir
 in half of the seasoning mixture and cook for 4 minutes.

5. Add string beans, yellow summer squash, and remaining seasoning mixture. Continue stir-frying the vegetables for 5 more
 minutes, or until the potatoes are cooked through and most (if
 not all) of the seasoning liquid has evaporated. Add the tofu,
 red pepper, and the remaining tablespoon of soy. Toss to mix,
 and stir-fry for 2 minutes. Transfer to a large serving bowl.

Kiriboshi Daikon with Shiitake Mushrooms and Tofu

SERVES 4

Kiriboshi are spaghettilike strips of dried and shredded daikon; they are sold in plastic bags in the Asian food section of supermarkets and at Japanese grocery stores. Rubbing the kiriboshi with a little salt helps break down the fibers and encourages hydration. If you use fresh daikon, which is also an option for this recipe, skip this step. The kiriboshi (or fresh daikon) simmers in a sweet soy broth with carrots and mushrooms to create a homey, comforting side dish popular throughout Japan. While it's delicious hot, it also tastes wonderful cold.

This recipe calls for using a drop-lid, or otoshi buta, which is a low-tech device for simmering. Simmering happens a lot in my mother's Tokyo kitchen, with vegetables, meat, and fish. A Japanese drop-lid is flat and made of wood, and instead of resting on top of the pot like a conventional lid, it sits directly on the ingredients inside. By staying so close to the food, it rechannels the broth through all the ingredients, maximizing the natural flavors of the food. A drop-lid should be a bit smaller than the diameter of the pot interior.

Otoshi buta drop-lids are hard to find in stores outside of Japan, but look for one at a store that carries Japanese cooking tools, or order it from a Web site like www.katagiri.com. Alternatively, you can fashion a substitute with aluminum foil. Cut a double layer of aluminum foil in a circle a bit smaller than the interior of your pot or pan, and lay it on top of the food you're simmering. When a pot is too small for my drop-lid, I use this method. It works just fine.

1 ounce kiriboshi daikon (thin strips of dried daikon), or
   1 1/4 cups of fresh daikon, shredded
1 3/4 teaspoons salt
One 3-x-5-inch rectangle of usu-age tofu (thin-fried
   tofu)
1 tablespoon canola oil or rice bran oil
5 shiitake mushrooms, stems cut off, and caps thinly
   sliced
1/3 cup matchsticks of carrot
1 1/2 cups dashi (page 52) for kiriboshi; if using fresh
   daikon, 2 1/2 cups
1 teaspoon granulated sugar
2 teaspoons sake
1 teaspoon reduced-sodium soy sauce

1. Place the kiriboshi in a bowl and gently rub with 1 teaspoon of the salt, as if you were washing socks. Rinse the kiriboshi and soak in a medium bowl of cold water, according to package directions, until tender, about 15 minutes. Saving the soaking liquid, transfer the hydrated kiriboshi to another bowl.
2. Bring a small saucepan of water to a boil. Add the usu-age tofu and simmer over medium heat, turning occasionally, for 1 minute; drain (this will remove excess oil). Cut the usu-age tofu lengthwise in half, and slice each half into thin strips.

3. Heat the oil over medium heat in a medium-size cooking pot equipped with a drop-lid or an aluminum foil equivalent. When the oil is hot, add the mushrooms, carrot, and kiriboshi (or fresh daikon) and sauté for 5 minutes. Add 1 cup of the reserved daikon soaking liquid and 1½ cups of the dashi (or 2½ cups of dashi if using fresh daikon) and bring the mixture to a boil.

4. Reduce the heat to medium-low, and stir in the fried tofu, along with the remaining ¾ teaspoon salt and the sugar, sake, and soy. Place a drop-lid over the ingredients and simmer, stirring occasionally, until the vegetables have absorbed all the liquid, about 20 minutes. Transfer to a serving dish.

———

Naomi's Gyoza Dumplings

SERVES 4

Loaded with vegetables and a bit of lean meat, these juicy Japanese pot stickers pack a lot of flavor into a little package.

This was one of the first dishes my mother taught me to make when I was young. Sitting side by side with my mom, I learned how to pack just the right amount of filling into each dumpling and carefully pinch the wrapper closed. My gyoza dumplings have more vegetables and less meat than my mother's version, and sometimes I make them completely vegetarian. The shiitake mushrooms have such a meaty texture and great flavor that I don't really need a whole lot of meat.

Nira is a member of the chive family, and is also known as Chinese chive or garlic chive. The green leaves are flat, unlike the round chives commonly sold in the U.S. I like their bold flavor— stronger than that of onions, but subtler than garlic—and the way they complement the sweet flavor of Napa cabbage. Nira also makes a great ingredient for stir-fry dishes. You can find both Nira and gyoza wrappers at Japanese grocery stores or markets like Whole Foods; another option is to use wonton wrappers.

This is a very child-friendly recipe: kids enjoy both making and eating these stuffed treats.

> 1/4 pound extra lean ground beef (sirloin)
> 1 cup finely chopped Napa cabbage
> 3 shiitake mushrooms, stems cut off, caps minced
> 1/2 bunch nira (Chinese chives), finely chopped (or 1/2 cup finely chopped chives)
> 2 scallions, roots cut off, minced
> Pinch of salt and freshly ground black pepper
> 24 round gyoza dumpling wrappers
> 2 tablespoons canola oil or rice bran oil
> 1 cup boiling water
> Reduced sodium-soy sauce, to use at the table
> Rice vinegar, to use at the table
> Hot pepper oil, to use at the table

1. Place the beef in a large bowl. Add the cabbage, mushrooms, nira, and scallions. Season the filling with several generous pinches of salt and grinds of pepper. Use your hands to blend the ingredients together.
2. Line a baking sheet with aluminum foil or parchment paper.

3. Fill a small bowl with cold water. For each dumpling, place 2 teaspoons of filling in the center of a gyoza wrapper. Then lightly dip one finger in the bowl and use it to trace around the inside of the gyoza wrapper, which will make it sticky enough to seal. Fold the wrapper in half with the edge on top. Gently press the edges from right to left to seal the dumpling, while pinching and folding every 1/4 inch of the edge facing you to make zigzag patterns. Place the dumpling on the baking sheet with the crimped side up. Continue making the dumplings in this manner until you have used up all the wrappers and filling.

4. Place a skillet large and deep enough to hold the dumplings over high heat. Add the 2 tablespoons of oil. When hot, reduce the heat to medium-low and add the dumplings, crimped side up. Cook the dumplings, uncovered, until they are lightly browned on the bottom, about 4 minutes.

5. Pour the boiling water into the skillet. Cover and steam-cook the dumplings over medium heat for 8 to 10 minutes, adding a tad more water as necessary, until the tops of the dumplings are translucent and all the water has evaporated. (If the tops turn translucent before all the water has evaporated, remove the cover and continue cooking the dumplings until the water is gone.) Lay out 4 plates and transfer 6 dumplings to each plate, with the golden bottoms facing up.

6. To serve, give each diner a small condiment dish, and let each person make his or her own dipping sauce to taste by mixing a tablespoon of soy, a splash of rice vinegar, and a few drops of hot pepper oil (if desired) in the dish.

Kinpira—Burdock and Carrot

SERVES 4

Kinpira is one of the classic Japanese home-cooked dishes, featuring two great root vegetables, burdock and carrots. In this sautéed dish the burdock combines beautifully with the sweet carrots, red peppers, and roasted sesame seeds. Crunchy, soft, sweet, and hot, no wonder this recipe is a popular winter dish in Japan.

Burdock, or gobo, is a fiber-rich Japanese root vegetable with a delectable earthiness. Look for burdock at Japanese markets or gourmet supermarkets.

    1 medium (8 ounce) burdock root
    1 tablespoon canola oil or rice bran oil
    2 dried Japanese (or Thai chili, Santaka, or Szechuan)
      red peppers
    1 cup carrot, cut into matchstick-size slivers
    1 tablespoon sake
    1 tablespoon reduced-sodium soy sauce
    2 teaspoons mirin
    1 teaspoon granulated sugar
    1 teaspoon toasted and ground sesame seeds

1. Scrub the exterior of the burdock root with a vegetable brush to remove excess dirt and the skin. Cut the burdock root into 2½- to 3-inch-long matchsticks, and rinse quickly under cold

water. You will have approximately 2 cups of burdock root matchsticks.

2. Heat the oil in a medium skillet over medium-high heat. Add the red peppers and sauté for 30 seconds. Add the burdock root and sauté until tender, about 3 minutes; it will appear translucent on the surface. Stir in the carrot and sauté for 2 minutes.

3. Reduce the heat to low and add the sake, soy, mirin, and sugar. Stir the vegetables for 1 minute more to allow them to absorb the sauce. Remove and discard the red peppers and arrange the vegetables in a mound in the center of a serving bowl and garnish with the sesame seeds.

Tokyo Salad

SERVES 4

Salads in Japan are a relatively modern phenomenon. However, sometimes modern is good, such as in this lively herb-filled medley of greens splashed with a light sesame dressing. Most mesclun salad mixes contain mizuna, a feathery Japanese green that adds an invigorating snap. Enjoy this salad during the warmer months.

½ pound pencil-thin asparagus, woody stem ends
   snapped off
6 cups mixed baby greens
½ cup thinly sliced celery
½ cup diced red bell pepper

1 scallion, roots and coarse portion of the tops cut off,
   and thinly sliced
2 tablespoons minced cilantro, plus 4 tiny sprigs for garnish
5 shiso leaves, thinly sliced
1 plum tomato, cored and cut into 12 wedges

Dressing

3 tablespoons rice vinegar
2 tablespoons minced red onion
1 teaspoon light brown sugar
1 tablespoon toasted sesame oil
Pinch of salt and freshly ground black pepper

1. Put 1 cup water in a medium skillet and bring to a boil. Add the asparagus and cook over high heat for 45 seconds, or until a sharp knife easily slides through one stem end. Drain and refresh under cold water. Transfer the asparagus to a plate lined with a double thickness of paper towels and let cool. Cut each spear diagonally into 1-inch-long pieces. Set aside several asparagus tips for the garnish.

2. Combine the cooked asparagus, greens, celery, red pepper, scallion, minced cilantro, and shiso in a salad bowl. Gently toss to mix.

3. In a small bowl, whisk together the vinegar, red onion, and brown sugar until the sugar is dissolved. Whisk in the sesame oil and season with a generous pinch of salt and several grinds of pepper. Pour the dressing over the salad and gently toss to mix. Lay out 4 salad plates. Arrange a portion of salad on each plate and garnish with 3 tomato wedges, the reserved asparagus tips, and the cilantro sprigs.

THE THIRD PILLAR: RICE

There was another Tokyo food vendor who pedaled through the streets of my childhood. Unlike the sweet potato man, he didn't sing a song. He attracted customers by parking his cart and switching on his equipment. His machine made a "crackle and pop" that rippled through the neighborhood and triggered throngs of kids to surround him with handfuls of rice.

He was the Rice Cracker Man, or Mr. Ponsenbei. *"Pon"* means "pop," and *"senbei"* means "rice cracker."

Mr. Ponsenbei took your handful of rice, poured it into a kind of waffle-iron machine powered by water pressure, and closed the lid. We would squeal with anarchic delight as the rice popped. A few seconds later what emerged from his machine was a thick, steaming hot, crunchy-moist fresh rice cake. It was so delicious—and only ten yen (about nine cents).

Like most Japanese mothers, the moms in our neighborhood were pretty strict about limiting sweets and snacks, but rice crackers were relatively healthy, and definitely on

Mom's approved list. Today, my mother declares, with the conviction of a Ph.D. in nutrition, "Rice is a good carbohydrate."

In Japan, rice is not just a nutritional pillar, it's an artistic ideal. Japanese people have an almost mystical connection with rice. "For the Japanese," wrote historian Amanda Mayer Stinchecum, "the vibrant green midsummer paddy fields, the ripened heads of grain bending the golden stalks at harvest time, the brown sheaves drying in the autumn sunlight symbolize wealth, fruition, prosperity."

You can think of Japan, along with much of the rest of Asia, as the world's biggest, longest-running rice party, a party that's been going on for about 1,300 years.

If you were a traveler back in Old Japan, say A.D. 900 or so, you would probably have carried a pouch of hoshii with you on the forest path. Hoshii was rice that was steamed, then dried, and carried in your pack. You added boiling water and, presto—instant trail food.

Rice is the staff of life and a constant companion, and it is served almost every day from childhood to the golden years. The Japanese turn rice grains into religious offerings, meals, treats, cooking oil, vinegar, and sake wine, and rice plant stems into tatami mats, paper, hats, ropes, and even, in the old days, sandals and blankets.

But rice is first and foremost a staple of home cooking. It is a food that is placed in its own special bowl and served as a feature of almost every meal, and usually served plain: no oil, no butter, no sauce.

"Don't leave a grain in your rice bowl," Japanese kids are

And above all there is rice. A glistening black lacquer rice cask set off in a dark corner is both beautiful to behold and a powerful stimulus to the appetite. Then the lid is briskly lifted, and this pure white freshly boiled food, heaped in its black container, each and every grain gleaming like a pearl, sends forth billows of warm steam—here is a sight no Japanese can fail to be moved by. Our cooking depends on shadows and is inseparable from darkness.

—Junichiro Tanizaki, In Praise of Shadows

constantly implored by their parents, "because farmers worked hard to grow it." As a result, after a meal, the typical Japanese rice bowl looks like a cat licked it clean. Leaving even one grain behind is such bad manners, it's practically a sin.

Japanese people most like to eat short-grain white rice, and they like it because it is chewy, a bit sticky and fluffy. The grains should stick together without being at all gummy. My mother's favorite rice is also Japan's favorite, the premium short-grain rice variety called Koshihikari. It has a superior texture and flavor—slightly sweet, the way we like our rice to taste.

One festive variety of rice, called mochi rice, is a highlight of the New Year's celebration, which is an even bigger extravaganza in Japan than in the West. Our New Year's festivities last seven days, beginning on the first of January—a week of celebration that culminates in Osechi, which is Japan's most festive annual family holiday meal. New Year's week is almost like Christmas, Thanksgiving, and the Fourth of July rolled into one. Everyone gets together, and I mean everyone—grandparents, aunts and uncles, cousins, neighbors, and close friends—to party and partake in special Osechi dishes, and to wish one another health, happiness, and prosperity throughout the new year.

The New Year's celebration is such a big production that, like everyone else in Japan, my mother starts shopping and cooking for it two weeks ahead of time. She goes to the Tsukiji market for the fish, the Ueno neighborhood market for dried foods, local markets for vegetables, and the local liquor shop to order cases of beer and bottles of sake. When my sister, Miki, and I still lived at home, we pitched in by helping cut and prepare some of the key ingredients, and so did our dad. It was something we all did together, because it was too much for any one person—even my mom.

In late December, a big event occurs in preparation for the New Year's celebration in homes throughout Japan. It is the backyard spectacle of "pounding the mochi," which transforms the rice into a fun, sticky-and-gooey treat that has the texture and consistency of pizza dough or bread dough. This Japanese tradition might appear a bit bizarre to the uninitiated outsider, so I'll explain.

In the mochi-pounding ritual, a group of grown men—including the father of the family—stand around a wooden tub filled with just-cooked rice that is still so hot it's steaming. The men take turns smacking the rice with a ceremonial mallet as they exclaim, "*Yoi-sho!*" which is loosely translatable as

"Let's go!" After each smack of the mallet, a woman reaches into the wooden tub to turn the mochi so that it will be pounded thoroughly and evenly, then pulls her hand out just in time for the mallet to come down again. The children love watching this spectacle, and there's lots of excitement as the mochi rice is gradually transformed into one large wad of thick gooey dough. A mallet-wielding mochi-smacking dad is just as much fun to a Japanese kid as a father wearing an apron and chef's hat at a backyard barbecue is to an American kid. But the mochi ritual has an almost sacramental dimension to it, even if that is not what is on the minds of the children.

"The Japanese believe that pounding rice brings out its sacred power, and that mochi contains the grain's spiritual essence," wrote Victoria Abbott Riccardi in *Untangling My Chopsticks: A Culinary Sojourn in Kyoto.* "In the olden days, farmers used to drop mochi down their wells as an offering to the Shinto god of water. Ten days later, they would scatter more mochi in their yards. If the crows pecked it up, legend had it the year would bring a good harvest."

When the pounded mochi has arrived at a taffylike consistency, it is divided into bite-size patties, or 2-inch-square cakes—and it's then ready to be eaten with a variety of seasonings like soy sauce, grated daikon, and soybean flour mixed with sugar. The mochi seasoned in soy sauce gets wrapped in nori seaweed. Mochi, eaten plain, has the same earthy, sweet flavor that short-grain rice has. The major difference is its chewy, gooey texture.

Throughout the New Year's holiday, we eat mochi instead

of regular rice. Special mochi-based dishes for the holiday season often include ozoni, a dashi-based clear soup with grilled mochi, small pieces of chicken, and mitsuba. On the last day of the holiday week, after six days of partying and eating all of the celebratory food, we give our stomachs a rest by sipping a rice porridge with seven seasonal herbs. So rice is both part of the festivity and an antidote to some of its excesses.

For many years rice has been the backbone of the high-carbohydrate diet consumed by the world's longest-lived people, Japanese women. Is there a connection between rice and obesity, and rice and longevity? Experts have many theories on the benefits of carbohydrates—which include, of course, not just rice, but vegetables and fruit.

One benefit has to do with the effect of carbohydrates on weight. "Long term, the studies show that people who keep weight off are people who eat a high-carbohydrate diet," according to Joanne Slavin, a professor of nutrition at the University of Minnesota who reviewed carbohydrate and whole grains research for the 2005 U.S. Dietary Guidelines Committee. I really think that rice is one of the main reasons that Japanese are relatively thin: two small bowls of rice at each meal is considered standard in Japan. The rice is eaten with other dishes—a few bites of rice, then fish, then some more rice, then veggies, then soup, then rice. This is how we fill ourselves up, leaving less room for jumbo desserts.

Rice has a number of nutritional benefits too. It is a rich source of complex carbohydrates, contains respectable amounts of certain key nutrients, and has little or no sodium, saturated fat, trans fat, or cholesterol. One researcher who strongly praises rice is Dr. Toshiie Sakata, deputy director of the Japanese Society for the Study of Obesity, who says rice "is an almost complete foodstuff—it is perfect nutritionally and sticky enough to chew."

The 2005 U.S. Dietary Guidelines pointed out the importance of carbohydrates in a healthy diet, suggesting that 45 to 65 percent of the daily calories consumed in a day by most adults should be from carbohydrates. In Japan, people get 60 percent of their daily calories from carbohydrates, an amount in accordance with the American guidelines, and rice accounts for about half of this.

Here's a tip for how you can eat even healthier than the average Japanese and capitalize on the chorus of expert advice to "eat more whole grains": eat brown rice!

I think you'll find rice, both white and brown, to be a simple, delicious addition to your diet, especially as a filling, natural replacement for any number of less nutritious alternatives.

Chicken and Eggs over Rice

SERVES 4

It's hard to beat this scrumptious combination of chicken, eggs, rice, and savory cooked negi. It's a very popular dish in Japan and for good reason: it's easy to make, extremely satisfying, and healthy.

Tokyo negi, found in many Japanese dishes, is like leek, but more tender and milder. However, you can substitute leek for the Tokyo negi if necessary and the dish will still be wonderful.

4 large eggs

1 cup dashi (page 52)

¼ cup sake

1 medium yellow onion, peeled, halved, and cut into thin crescents

1 Tokyo negi (or 1 small leek) roots and rough portion of the top cut off, cleaned, rinsed, and cut diagonally into thin slices

½ teaspoon reduced-sodium soy sauce

1 teaspoon granulated sugar

1 teaspoon salt

1 teaspoon mirin

½ pound boneless, skinless chicken breasts, cut into bite-size pieces

6 cups hot cooked brown or white rice (page 54)

4 sprigs mitsuba (or Italian parsley)

1. Break the eggs into a medium bowl and whisk until just mixed.
2. Place the dashi and sake in a medium saucepan over high heat. Add the onion and Tokyo negi (or leek) and bring the mixture to a boil. Reduce the heat to medium and simmer until the vegetables are tender, about 5 minutes. Stir in the soy, sugar, salt, and mirin.
3. Stir in the chicken pieces and cook for 3 minutes. Pour the beaten eggs over the surface of the chicken mix, so that the egg forms a sort of "cap." Reduce the heat to low and cook the mixture for approximately 2 minutes, or until the egg and chicken are cooked through. Stir the mixture and turn off the heat.
4. Lay out 4 large bowls. Fill each one with 1 ½ cups of hot cooked rice and ladle one fourth of the chicken-egg mixture over the top. Garnish each serving with a sprig of mitsuba (or parsley).

Japanese Comfort Food: Rice Balls

SERVES 4 (3 RICE BALLS PER PERSON)

Rice balls are the quintessential Japanese comfort food. At my grandparents' farmhouse in the Japanese countryside, my grandmother always kept a plate of fresh rice balls on the kitchen table. Neighbors and family members who dropped by throughout the day would grab a rice ball and pop it in their mouth. My mother made rice balls for our school lunch boxes and family picnics. Today, you can join the millions of Japanese who regularly enjoy rice balls (they call them onigiri or omusubi) as a light meal or healthy on-the-go snack.

This recipe calls for three different fillings for the rice balls. One of the fillings, umeboshi (pickled and dried Japanese apricots, which for some reason are often labeled as plums in the United States), is the number one filling for rice balls, and the most popular companion for a bed of rice in lunch boxes throughout Japan. You can find them in the Asian food section of supermarkets, in Japanese grocery stores, and at online stores like Eden Foods, or by searching other online shopping sites.

Please note, once you make all the rice balls, unless you label them, you won't be able to tell what's inside. However, growing up, this was part of the fun; I never knew what filling I might encounter when I bit into a rice ball!

2 ounces salmon fillet

$\frac{1}{16}$ ounce small bonito flakes

$1\frac{1}{2}$ teaspoons reduced-sodium soy sauce

4 pitted umeboshi

6 cups cooked brown or white rice (page 54)

Six 8-inch square sheets toasted nori (sea vegetable),
   each cut into four squares

1. Preheat a grill or a broiler to medium. Place the salmon on the grill, or on a foil-lined baking sheet, and grill or broil for 6 to 7 minutes, or until the salmon is just cooked through. Let cool. Remove the skin from the salmon and break the salmon into 4 pieces.

2. Mix the bonito flakes with the soy in a small bowl.

3. Place the umeboshi in a small bowl.

4. Fill a medium bowl with cold water. Lightly wet both hands to

prevent rice grains from sticking to your palms. Place ½ cup of rice in one hand and use the thumb of your other hand to make a deep indentation in the center of the rice. Place a piece of salmon in the indentation and then cover it over with the rice. Lightly squeeze both hands around the rice to shape it into a round that looks like a smaller and fatter hamburger patty, rotating and gently squeezing the rice a couple of times until it becomes well packed and solid. Repeat process with the other 3 pieces of salmon, dipping your hands into the cold water between the making of each rice ball.

5. Continue forming the rice balls in the same manner, using a quarter of the portion of the soy-seasoned bonito flakes per rice ball until you have 4 bonito-filled rice balls. When the bonito flake mixture is gone, make the final 4 rice balls with the umeboshi in the center. You will now have 12 rice balls, which you can choose to label or not—depending on whether you and your family like surprises.

6. For each rice ball, put a square of nori in your palm, on top of which you lay the rice ball with one of the flat sides down. Press the corners of the nori over the rice. Place another square of nori over the top of the rice ball, and press the corners down over the exposed rice. Gently squeeze the rice ball with both hands to ensure that the nori adheres firmly to the rice. Continue wrapping the remaining rice balls in the same manner. And that's it—they are now ready to be eaten.

Tokyo Kitchen Tips

Use freshly cooked rice that is still warm or even hot to create the best-tasting rice balls.

When shaping it into balls, give the rice a moderate squeeze, not too hard and not too gentle. The rice should be packed just firmly enough so that it does not fall apart before it reaches your mouth.

———

Beef over Rice

SERVES 4

Here's a perfect example of how Japanese home cooks create a delicious and filling beef dish—with very small portions of beef. An abbreviated version of sukiyaki (a combination of thinly sliced beef and vegetables in a sweet soy broth), this is spooned over hot cooked rice in a bowl.

Thinly sliced beef is available in the freezer section of most Japanese markets. It's convenient to use, extremely tender, and perfect for this hearty cold-weather dish. If you choose to purchase the beef in a regular market, freeze the meat before you cut it. This will enable you to carve it (with an extremely sharp knife) into paper-thin slices.

I often think that the best part of this beef bowl isn't the beef, but the hot nutty rice saturated with the sweet beef juices.

2 cups dashi (page 52)
¼ cup sake

1 medium yellow onion, peeled, halved, and cut into
  thin crescents
1 Tokyo negi (or 1 small leek), with roots and rough portion of the top cut off, cleaned, rinsed, and cut diagonally into thin slices
3 tablespoons reduced-sodium soy sauce
1 tablespoon granulated sugar
1 teaspoon fine-ground sea salt
1 teaspoon mirin
½ pound very thinly sliced beef fillet (about ⅛ inch
  thick), or, if you prefer, ground beef
6 cups hot cooked brown or white rice (page 54)
1 scallion, roots and top portion cut off, and thinly sliced

1. Place the dashi and sake in a medium saucepan over high heat.
   Add the onion and Tokyo negi (or leek) and bring the mixture
   to a boil. Reduce the heat to medium and simmer until the
   vegetables are tender, about 5 minutes. Stir in the soy, sugar,
   salt, and mirin. Add the beef and simmer until it is just cooked
   through, about 40 seconds (it will cook rapidly if cut into paper-
   thin slices).
2. Lay out 4 bowls. Fill each one with 1½ cups of hot cooked rice
   and ladle even portions of the beef mixture over the top.
   Garnish each serving with a sprinkling of scallion.

THE FOURTH PILLAR: SOY

It is August, and my husband, Billy, and I are lounging on the porch of our rented apartment in the Aoyama neighborhood of Tokyo.

Summers in Tokyo can be a mind-blasting experience, with stratospheric heat and humidity making the long distances between buildings and subway stations seem like endless walks. Everybody sinks into a kind of waking coma, yearning for refreshment at the end of the day. Tonight we are sitting in lawn chairs, waiting for a cool breeze.

I'm clinging to a cold Asahi beer.

On the table in front of us is a bamboo basket full of boiled fresh green soybeans, or edamame, chilled and sprinkled with a little salt. A bit of salt tastes great after a long sweaty day and a bath, especially when added to the pure natural taste of the soybean in its pod form.

I slowly squeeze a pod between my index finger and thumb to push a bean loose. As soon as the edge of the bean is out, I bring it to my lips and squeeze the pod harder to pop it into my mouth. Sliding my fingers up the pod, I repeat the squeezing and popping motions two more times, until each of the three beans that are usually in a pod have been eaten.

———

Whenever I hold a handful of soybeans, I think of hot summer nights, because for as long as I can remember, the combination of edamame and cold beer has been like a national pastime for Japanese in the summer.

When I was a young salarywoman in Tokyo, they were part of our afterwork ritual. As soon as we left the office, my colleagues and I would head for a beer garden on a department store rooftop. I can picture it now.

The beer garden is a casual bar-restaurant with benches, communal tables, and rows of lanterns hanging in the air. Walking in, we take over a table, and as soon as we are seated we order edamame and pitchers of draft beer—first things first. At a place like this, beer mugs are uncharacteristically large for Japan. The men take off their jackets, loosen their ties, and roll up their shirtsleeves. A cool wind brushes our faces.

The neon signs of Ginza flicker and illuminate the night, and even at 10 P.M. some of the surrounding office building windows are still lit, with salarymen hard at work at tiny desks pushed against one another.

Our laughter climbs up into the sky and drifts away on the breeze.

———

Tonight, on the back porch of our apartment in Tokyo, I toss an empty edamame pod into a bowl placed next to the bamboo basket. Reaching for another pod, and another after that, I keep going until the basket is empty and the bowl is piled high with empty pods. Soon it will be time for dinner. And now another memory surfaces.

I hear a voice from my childhood. My mother's.
In the thick of preparations for dinner, she is calling me into the kitchen with a request: "Naomi, please go get two pieces of silken tofu. Here are some yen."

The tofu store, or tofu-ya, was four blocks away from our house.

In the days before mega-supermarkets, we bought most of our food from neighborhood shops, each with its own specialty: a vegetable and fruit store, a fish store, a meat shop, a rice store, and a bakery. Japan was, and to some extent still is, a nation of small, family-owned stores, where you might find three generations working behind the counter.

The tofu store, too, was family-run, and they made fresh handmade tofu on the premises. It was like a butcher shop, only for tofu, or soybean curd. I would walk over to the store with my mother's red shopping basket and be greeted by the husband and wife proprietors. Both wore white-cotton bandannas on their heads, rubber aprons, and rainboots, and had rolled up their shirtsleeves.

Two big square pools of water dominated the store: one pool for blocks of silken (very delicate) tofu, and the other for cotton (firm) tofu. There were glass display cases for broiled tofu and for fried age (pronounced "*ah*-gay") tofu, thin and thick. There were also tofu patties, sheets of soymilk skin (*yuba*), and a huge steaming container of leftover soy fiber and protein (*okara*).

I'd belly up to the counter and say, *"Kinugoshi tofu wo nicho, kudasai."* ("May I have two blocks of silken tofu, please.")

The shop lady would grab a plastic container in her left hand, dip her right hand into the pool, reach for a block of tofu, scoop it up ever so gently so as not to break it, and as soon as it was out of the water, flip it into the container.

The tofu store wasn't the only place to buy fresh tofu. There also used to be "tofu men" who bicycled through the back-streets of Tokyo.

You would hear the sound of the tofu man's flute around 4 P.M., when people were starting to prepare dinner. You brought out your own bowl and he served you chilled tofu straight from the box in his pull cart. I haven't seen a tofu man on a bike for a long time. And tofu stores are becoming less common too. These days, most people in Japan buy packaged tofu in the supermarket, just as people do in the United States.

———

In Japan, a day without eating some form of the almighty, low-calorie, low-fat, high-protein soybean—mainly in the form of miso soup, a chunk of sliced tofu, soy sauce, or some sticky fermented natto beans—is almost unthinkable. At some Japanese tables, three or more soy products might be served in the same meal.

My father, Shigeo, calls soy "protein from the fields," and my mother—ever the nutrition expert—declares that soy "is a fabulous source of protein to replace meat." Which is quite true. Part of what she loves about soy is its versatility. As she notes, "You can use tofu in miso soup, make chilled tofu, put tofu in nabe [a one-pot stew], or simmer atsu-age [thick-fried] tofu with vegetables."

Tofu found its way to Japan from China about a thousand years ago, and soon became one of the favorite protein dishes of vegetarian Zen Buddhist priests, especially in the old capital of Kyoto, which has been a hotbed of tofu production ever since. In Kyoto today, you can still visit exquisite tofu-themed restaurants like Okutan, which opened for business in 1635. The menu there features simmered tofu, sesame tofu, vegetable tempura, grated yam, and tofu baked and coated with miso and pepper leaf buds.

Miso, the fermented paste mixture of cooked soybeans with rice or wheat or barley, also made the leap over from China, but it arrived even earlier than tofu, perhaps around A.D. 700. The different flavors of miso have inspired adjectives like rich, complex, buttery, nutty, sweet, meaty, robust, and earthy. This range of tastes gives miso a place of honor in every Japanese kitchen as a savory seasoning ingredient for soups, marinades, sautéing sauces, grilling sauces, soup broths, and garnishes.

Japan's first best-selling cookbook, published in Osaka way back in 1782, was *Tofu Hyakuchin* (*100 Tofu Recipes*). The book was so successful that it spawned a sequel a year later, *100 More Tofu Recipes*. The original book featured chapters called "In the Know Recipes," "Odd and Creative Recipes," "Ultimate Best Recipes," and "Tofu Tidbits." The very first recipe in *100 Tofu*

Recipes is tofu broiled with miso paste—a dish that has two soy products in one!

Soy has recently been the subject of a deluge of positive press in the medical and scientific world, culminating in the United States with the Food and Drug Administration's approval in 1999 of the health claim: "Diets low in saturated fat and cholesterol that include 25 grams of soy protein a day may reduce the risk of heart disease." This position was echoed by Britain's Food Standards Agency.

In 2001, the *Harvard Women's Health Watch* reported that "soybeans are unique among plant foods in supplying all the essential amino acids that the human body needs, making soy protein similar in quality to meat protein—but with largely unsaturated instead of saturated fat."

Some experts are convinced that Japan's relatively high consumption of soy products is a contributing factor to Japanese people's health and longevity. For example, Dr. Rudolph Tanzi of Harvard Medical School believes the high level of soy in the Japanese diet "provides forms of estrogen-like products that can be protective against Alzheimer's disease."

Other soy advocates point to the fact that Japanese women eat much more soy than people in the West, and have much lower rates of breast cancer, though there is no guarantee that these two facts are directly linked.

Moreover, the research on soy is not all positive. Though some studies have suggested that soy consumption can relieve menopausal symptoms and help prevent not just breast cancer and osteoporosis in women but prostate cancer in men, other studies have linked overconsumption of soy with an increased risk of breast cancer as well as of thyroid and fertility problems.

Unfortunately, most of the research on soy, both positive and negative, is based on samples that are too small to be statistically significant, on population comparisons, or on animal studies that have not been confirmed in human trials. "There have been no double-blind controlled studies, the gold standard in scientific research, looking at the safety of soy in humans," noted the *New York Times* in 2004, "and what research there is has produced conflicting results, providing little guidance and creating a heated debate among experts." The *Times* did report that no studies on humans have concluded that soy causes breast cancer in women.

According to several experts, soy is a great food choice when consumed in moderation. Mindy S. Kurzer, a nutrition professor at the University of Minnesota, for example, believes that "soy foods are great; they appear to be absolutely safe when consumed at levels consumed in Asia, which is one to two servings a day." The *Harvard Health Watch* concluded that "soy foods are best viewed as a good protein source to include in a healthy, balanced diet that is low in saturated fats and includes a mix of proteins, vegetables, fruits, and whole grains."

George L. Blackburn, associate professor of nutrition at Harvard Medical School, believes that soy's benefits are part of an overall Asian-style diet and "soy lifestyle": portion control; eating fish, lean meat, poultry, and lots of vegetables; replacing some portions of milk or meat with soy; and exercise, such as bicycling and walking.

One thing is clear—the Japanese are the world-champion

soy eaters, consuming an average of up to 50 grams of soy per day, compared with 10 grams for the average Chinese and less than 5 grams for the average Westerner. And many Westerners who eat soy eat it much differently than the Japanese do. Japanese are mostly eating soy in its more natural and less processed forms—tofu, miso, edamame, and natto beans (an exception, of course, is soy sauce)—not in the soy supplements, soy shakes, soy burgers, tofu cheesecake, or soy energy bars that are so popular in the West.

Still, at least one form of natural soy is really catching on in the United States. At a cocktail party I attended not long ago in New York, I was delighted to see a huge bowl of edamame next to a platter of beautifully arranged cheeses. Edamame seems to have achieved "it" food status as a snack or appetizer. To see edamame beans become chic seems funny to me—it's as if the girl who grew up next door to us in Japan suddenly became a superstar.

And while it may not yet be easy to find fresh edamame, frozen edamame, both in and out of the pod, taste great, and are becoming more and more widely available.

At a Whole Foods Market recently, I saw a three-generation debate taking place in the frozen foods section. A five-year-old girl was pulling a package of frozen edamame out of the freezer display case. The girl's grandmother suggested, "Why don't we get French fries." The girl's mother intervened firmly, "*No!* We are not eating French fries for two weeks. We are getting edamame instead!"

Just maybe, I thought, I'm watching a snapshot of food history: past, present, and future.

Clear Soup with Tofu and Shiitake Mushrooms

SERVES 4

Clear soups epitomize the pure, simple elegance of Japanese home cooking. They often appear on special occasions, such as for New Year's. The broth consists of first-quality dashi seasoned with salt and a touch of soy to give it a pretty amber tint. The added ingredients tend to be delicate and small in quantity in order to underscore the sophisticated beauty of this dish.

> One 8-ounce block silken tofu
> 4 shiitake mushroom caps, thinly sliced
> 4 cups dashi (page 52)
> 2 teaspoons reduced-sodium soy sauce
> 1 1/2 teaspoons salt
> 1 teaspoon sake
> 1 scallion, roots and rough portion of the top cut off,
>   and thinly sliced

1. Place the tofu in a colander or strainer and gently rinse under cold water.
2. Bring a small saucepan of water to a boil. Reduce the heat to medium-low, add the tofu, and gently simmer for 2 minutes. Drain, and dice the tofu into small pieces.
3. Bring another small saucepan of water to a boil. Add the sliced

shiitake caps and simmer over low heat for 3 minutes, or until tender. Drain.

4. Bring the dashi to a boil in a large saucepan. Stir in the soy, salt, and sake.

5. Lay out 4 small soup bowls. In each bowl, arrange a portion of tofu cubes on one side of the bottom of the bowl and a cluster of the sliced shiitake caps on the other. Gently pour the dashi into each bowl, trying not to disturb the arranged ingredients, and garnish with the scallion slices.

Tokyo Kitchen Tips

Use First Dashi (not Second Dashi) for your soup base for the best flavor.

Cooking the soup ingredients separately ensures a lovely clear (versus cloudy) broth.

———

Miso Soup with Daikon and Tofu

SERVES 4

I often use a combination of red and white miso because I like the bite of the red and the softness of the white together in the same dish. Usu-age tofu has an appealing meatiness, which, along with the tender daikon, gives this soup a nice heft. The daikon leaves add a lovely watery crunch. Most Japanese stores sell daikon with the leaves attached. However, if your daikon has no leaves, watercress's peppery-tasting leaves make a fine substitute.

One 3-x-5-inch rectangle usu-age tofu (thin-fried tofu)
6 cups dashi (page 52)
2 cups daikon, cut into matchstick-size slivers
Several daikon leaves (or small handful of watercress),
cut into thin ribbons
2 ½ tablespoons red or white miso (or use a combination of both)

1. Bring a small saucepan of water to a boil. Add the usu-age tofu
and gently simmer over medium heat, turning a few times, for
1 minute; drain (this will remove excess oil). Cut the usu-age
tofu in half lengthwise, and slice each half into thin strips. Set
aside.

2. Place the dashi in a medium saucepan. Add the daikon slivers
and bring the mixture to a boil. Cook until the daikon begins
to look translucent, about 5 minutes. Stir in the daikon leaves
(or watercress) and the usu-age tofu and bring the mixture
back to a boil. Reduce the heat to medium and cook for 2
minutes, or until the greens are tender. Gently whisk in the
miso and turn off the heat. Ladle the soup into 4 small bowls.

Tokyo Kitchen Tip

When boiling any hard-root vegetables, such as daikon, place the vegetables in a cold liquid (water or broth) and bring to a boil. This enables
the whole vegetable to cook evenly. If you place a hard vegetable in a
boiling liquid, by the time the core is tender, the exterior is overcooked.

Tasty Summer Edamame

SERVES 4

Nutty edamame are a popular accompaniment to cold beer. The fresh beans are available during the summer months at select stores and farmers markets in the United States. If you can't find fresh edamame, the frozen ones in the pods make a fine substitute.

Several branches fresh edamame (or one 16-ounce bag
frozen edamame in the pod)
Salt

1. For *fresh edamame*: Rinse the pods on their stalks under cold water to remove any residual dirt. Cut off any leaves and roots from the stalk. Bring a stockpot of water to a boil. Add the edamame, breaking the branches in half if necessary to fit in the pot. Simmer for 5 minutes or until the beans, when squeezed from their pod, are tender. Drain the edamame, rinse under cold water, and transfer to a serving bowl. Sprinkle with pinches of salt, toss, and let cool to room temperature.

2. For *frozen edamame*: Fill a large saucepan with several inches of water and bring to a boil. Add the edamame and cook, according to package directions, until tender. (Many brands of frozen edamame in the pods have been precooked, so they

will take much less time to become tender than the fresh soybeans.) Drain, rinse under cold water, and transfer to a serving bowl. Sprinkle with pinches of salt, toss, and let cool to
room temperature.

3. To eat, bring a pod to your mouth and gently squeeze the
beans out of their pods. Discard the pods in a separate dish.

THE FIFTH PILLAR: NOODLES

The prime minister of Japan was at home, sitting in a comfortable red chair. He was watching a jumbo television screen. And he was thinking about noodles.

It was August 4, 2005, and the shaggy-haired, opera-and-Elvis-loving prime minister, Junichiro Koizumi, was in the thick of political combat. Fighting the biggest battle of his career, he was trying to break up and privatize the Japanese national postal service, which is also the world's biggest financial institution, holding nearly $3 trillion (yes, that's *trillion*) in assets. That week, he was threatening to dissolve the Diet (the Japanese parliament) over the issue and call an election that could throw him and his party out of office.

But now, as he sat inside his dazzling, brand-new home-office complex on a hillside in the heart of Tokyo, the prime minister was taking time to consider a subject that was dear to his heart—the taste of instant ramen noodles in a pouch.

The head of the Japanese government is an ardent noodle connoisseur. He loves to slip out for a fast salaryman's lunch at crowded local Chinese-style ramen shops in his neighborhood, and he treated President George W. Bush to dinner at a Tokyo noodle restaurant when the Texan was in town. In New York in 2004, after throwing a perfect first pitch at Yankee Stadium, Koizumi ordered his motorcade to make a stop at the Nippon restaurant on East Fifty-second Street, where he packed away two servings of buckwheat soba noodles—one hot and one cold.

On this day in the summer of 2005 his focus was on noodles in outer space. Inside the U.S. space shuttle *Discovery,* 220 miles above Earth and traveling at 17,500 miles an hour, a forty-year-old Japanese astronaut named Soichi Noguchi was fielding a question from his boss in a live video linkup.

"Mr. Noguchi," asked Prime Minister Koizumi, "I tried the space noodles, but how did they taste in space? Were they good?"

The noodles in question were an experimental batch whipped up by the leading noodle conglomerate, Nissin Food Products Company, specifically for space travel. Dubbed "Space Ram" (for "ramen"), they were fried and vacuum-sealed in a thick spicy broth and came in four flavors: soy sauce, miso, curry, and pork.

The astronaut, who like the prime minister is an avid noodle lover, considered the question.

"Space noodles," replied Noguchi, "were one of the things I was really looking forward to." His verdict: "They were surprisingly close to the delicious taste of noodles on Earth."

Some 300 miles away from Tokyo, in Osaka Prefecture, the man who invented both instant noodles (in 1958) and Space

Ram (in 2005), a ninety-five-year-old named Momofuku Ando, could barely contain his emotions. "It's almost like a dream," said Ando, the founder of Nissin. "To think—ramen traveling up in space!"

———

Like Prime Minister Koizumi, Astronaut Noguchi, and tens of millions of other Japanese, I love noodles.

I love the textures of noodles, all kinds of noodles—soba, udon, ramen, somen, you name it.

I love their flavors.

I love their reliable, chewy character.

I love their casual, elegant nonchalance.

I love the way they look—for example, the elemental beauty of white udon noodles nestled in a rich brown broth, floating alongside green vegetables and a drifting piece of tofu, sending forth ribbons of intoxicating aroma from the bowl.

I love how different noodle dishes tell the stories of different seasons, especially winter and summer. The winter tale is told by clay-pot-cooked udon wheat noodles with vegetables and an egg and shrimp tempura in hot soup. The clay pot goes directly from the stove to the table, keeping the food very hot. I feel warmer inside from the very first spoonful.

In the thick of a steamy summer afternoon, when appetite and energy are at all-time lows, I cool off and energize with cold buckwheat soba noodles or Chinese egg noodle salad for lunch. Or I enjoy thin somen angel-hair-style noodles served over ice cubes in a shallow glass bowl with condiments like grated ginger, minced scallions, and wasabi. The super-thin noodles, garnished with a shiso leaf and floating over rocks of ice, remind me of a narrow stream flowing through the mountains. Just looking at it, I feel cooler.

My mother has her own summer favorites. "I like cold soba with tempura and garnishes," she says, "or cold Chinese noodles with five toppings, like sliced cucumbers, tomatoes, eggs, wakame seaweed, and ham. You can serve it with a dressing made of rice vinegar, soy sauce, and sesame oil, plus hot mustard."

My mother likes noodles in the form of spaghetti too. Sometimes she combines cod roe with spaghetti and garnishes the dish with strips of nori seaweed, in her own completely unique Japanization of pasta. Like many Japanese, she enjoys noodle dishes from both East and West. However, traditional Japanese noodles like udon and soba are never served with the cheese, cream, oil, or butter or tomato sauces that typically ac-

Last month I found my Japanese husband in the kitchen cooking hiyashi chuuka—cold ramen noodles with a sweet sauce, sliced cucumbers, tomatoes, and small sausages. A very quick meal for him to make, but a lifesaver to me. How he had guessed what a pregnant American woman wanted is beyond me!

Japan has reminded me that you should be thankful before and after you eat, which prepares your body to imbibe all the good of the meal—the food, the company, and the memory.

—Elise Tokumasu,
an American woman living in Tokyo

company Italian pasta. Cold soba noodles, for example, are usually served with just a basic dipping sauce.

There's also often an East-West difference in noodle-eating manners. Many Japanese, especially those who are over sixty, including our prime minister, Mr. Koizumi, slurp their noodles in the "old school" way. Older Japanese were trained practically since birth that it was chic to slurp both soup and noodles loudly, with maximum gusto, to show how much they were enjoying their food. As a member of the younger generation of Japanese, who are increasingly happy to enjoy their noodles discreetly, with a minimum of theatrics, I don't slurp. It's all a matter of which side of the generational noodle divide you're on.

There are no fewer than 200,000 noodle shops in Japan, more than any other kind of restaurant, and Japanese eat some 6 billion packets of instant ramen per year, dwarfing America's 2.6 billion. Many of Japan's noodle shops are real hole-in-the-wall joints—maybe ten seats, one counter, and a serve-yourself pitcher of water—but you can find noodle nirvana in even the most modest establishment.

According to food historian Naomichi Ishige, the roots of Japan's noodlemania are deep. "From documentary evidence," he wrote, "it is clear that in the mid-seventeenth century, soba was a low-class food, but in the early eighteenth century, splendidly-equipped soba shops emerged where persons of rank would eat, and in the late eighteenth century, senior samurai in attendance at the homes of daimyo [feudal lords] discussed which soba or sushi shops were the tastiest."

By one estimate, in 1818 there were more than 3,000 soba shops in Tokyo (or Edo, as it was then called), so many in such a small area that some of them were only fifty yards apart. Amazed visitors described the city as "soba crazy."

After the catastrophic great Tokyo earthquake and fire in 1923, Chinese noodle stands popped up amid the ruins, offering affordable ramen served in hearty beef, chicken, or fish stock, topped with pork and garnished with chopped onions and seaweed. A "ramen boom" was born, and ramen shops became the hamburger stands of Japan.

Today, local noodle shops in Tokyo and elsewhere make home deliveries on motorized scooters that carry vats of hot noodles and broth. Near train stations, you'll find a fast-food-in-a-hurry version of a soba restaurant called "tachiguisoba"—or "stand and eat soba"—where they serve you at a stand-up counter instead of at a table.

Japanese noodle preferences are often a function of where you grew up.

To the south and west of Tokyo, in places like Kyoto and Osaka, people prefer chubby white udon, wheat-flour noodles.

Like many people from Tokyo, I like soba, the thin, brownish, nutty-tasting noodle that is usually made from a blend of buckwheat and wheat flour. The higher the percentage of buckwheat, the better. Soba is also very popular among people in the cool north of Japan, where buckwheat is grown.

While the shape of most long strands of Italian pasta is tubular, soba is cut with four edges, which I think adds to its irresistibly tasty, chewy texture. It's often served in a little bamboo-surfaced lacquerware box, both at home and at restaurants, adding to its aesthetic appeal.

Soba noodles also have symbolic value in Japan. As midnight approaches on New Year's Eve, we have a tradition of eating buckwheat noodles that are called toshikoshi soba, or "Passing of the Year Noodles." The noodles are a symbol of new beginnings, new hope—and longevity.

Nutritionally, there's a lot to love about buckwheat, which is a good source of protein, fiber, whole grains, and complex carbohydrates.

———

The Perfect Bowl of Soba Noodles

SERVES 4

What can I say? The name captures it all. Buckwheat soba noodles and shrimp tempura in a flavorful authentic Japanese broth is my idea of perfection in a bowl, Tokyo-style. Shichimi togarashi is a seven-spice mix that adds a hot, spicy, peppery flavor to the broth. It is a distinctly Japanese blend of ground red pepper, roasted orange peel, white and black sesame seeds, Japanese pepper, seaweed, and ginger. You could use ground cayenne if you cannot find shichimi togarashi, but it will simply add a kick of heat to the noodles versus the burst of heat and flavor you get from the combination of seven spices.

4 cups dashi (page 52)
1 cup well-packed large bonito flakes
¼ cup sake
¼ cup mirin
¼ cup reduced-sodium soy sauce
1 teaspoon granulated sugar

1 teaspoon salt

8 pieces of shrimp tempura (page 143)

1 pound dried soba (thin buckwheat noodles)

1 scallion, roots and rough portion of the top cut off,
and thinly sliced

4 tiny sprigs mitsuba or Italian parsley

Shichimi togarashi (dried seven-spice chili mix, available
in any Japanese market)

1. Place the dashi in a large saucepan over high heat. Stir in the
bonito flakes and bring the mixture to a boil. Turn off the heat
and pour the dashi through a fine-mesh sieve lined with a double layer of cheesecloth to strain out the bonito flakes. Transfer
the dashi back to the saucepan and stir in the sake, mirin, soy,
sugar, and salt. Bring the mixture just to a boil, reduce the heat
to very low, and keep warm.

2. Place a large saucepan of water over medium-high heat for
cooking the soba.

3. Make the shrimp tempura according to the directions for tempura on page 143.

4. Bring a saucepan of water to a boil. Add the soba and stir to
prevent sticking. Cook the soba, according to package directions, until just cooked through. (Most soba cooks for 6 to 8
minutes, but test the noodles as they boil.) Drain them when
they are just past al dente. After draining, rinse the soba in a
colander under warm water to remove any residual starch.

5. Bring the dashi back to a boil. Lay out 4 large soup bowls and
distribute 4 even portions of noodles among the bowls. Lay 2
pieces of shrimp tempura per bowl over the noodles and pour
one fourth of the amount of dashi around the tempura in each

bowl. Garnish each serving with some scallion and a sprig of mitsuba. Let diners season their soup with some shichimi togarashi, as desired.

Tokyo Kitchen Tip

Estimate the shrimp tempura and soba cooking time so that both can be served immediately after cooked.

Cold Soba Buckwheat Noodles

SERVES 4

When the weather turns hot in Japan, this cool noodle dish becomes a refreshing lunch and dinner staple. It's nourishing, yet light. The sauce requires only three ingredients and is a snap to put together. However, if you want, you can buy a ready-made dipping sauce at any Japanese market. The sauces are usually marked "Dipping Sauce for Noodles—Ready to Use Soba Tsuyu" on the label. Of course, I think freshly made is best, but these ready-made sauces can be good.

Traditionally, the noodles are placed on a noodle basket (called a "zaru," which is why this dish is called "zaru soba" in Japan) or on a soba tray lined with a bamboo strainer for draining any excess water. While you can purchase such baskets and trays at stores featuring Japanese cooking items and tableware, it's not necessary. Simply make sure your noodles are well drained before mounding them onto the center of the plates.

2 cups dashi (page 52)

¹/₂ cup mirin

¹/₂ cup reduced-sodium soy sauce

12 ounces dried soba (thin buckwheat noodles)

¹/₂ cup finely grated daikon, excess liquid drained off

2 tablespoons toasted and ground white sesame seeds

Fresh grated wasabi (or from a tube)

1 scallion, roots and rough portion of the top cut off,
     and thinly sliced

One 8-inch square sheet of toasted nori (sea vegetable),
     snipped into short, thin ribbons

1. Combine the dashi, mirin, and soy in a medium saucepan over high heat. Bring to a boil, turn off the heat, and let cool to room temperature. (Or, to speed up chilling, place the cooled dipping sauce in a small metal bowl, nestle the small metal bowl in a larger bowl half filled with ice and water, and stir the sauce occasionally.) Pour the cooled sauce in a sauce pitcher and bring to the table.

2. When the dipping sauce is ready, bring a large saucepan of water to a boil. Add the soba and stir to prevent sticking. Cook the soba, according to package directions, until just cooked through, about 6 to 8 minutes. However, test the noodles as they boil and drain them when they are just past al dente. After draining, rinse the soba under cold water to chill them and eliminate any residual starch.

3. Mound the grated daikon on a small plate. Place the toasted sesame seeds in a small bowl with a small spoon for serving. Arrange a little mound of wasabi (about 2 teaspoons) on a small

plate along with the scallions. Bring all these garnishes to the table.

4. Arrange the soba on 4 soba trays lined with bamboo strainers (or 4 salad plates). Sprinkle the nori over the top of the soba and bring the noodles to the table, along with 4 small sauce bowls or cups. Let diners help themselves to approximately ½ cup dipping sauce each and then season it to their liking by topping with grated daikon, toasted sesame seeds, wasabi, and scallions.

———

Tamago—Japanese-Style Omelette

SERVES 4

This is a classic Japanese home-cooked classic side dish. How is it different from a Western-style omelette? For one, this omelette uses dashi instead of cheese. Second, it has a tiny bit of sugar to make it subtly sweet. Third, because of the cooking method, when you slice the omelette, the sides of the little egg "logs" will have a pattern that looks like the annual growth rings on a tree. Quite pretty! My mother often makes this tamago dish to go with cold soba noodles.

8 large eggs

2 tablespoons dashi (page 52)

1 teaspoon sake

½ teaspoon granulated sugar

½ teaspoon reduced-sodium soy sauce

Salt to taste

2 1/2 teaspoons canola oil or rice bran oil
1/4 cup finely grated daikon, excess liquid drained off
2 teaspoons freshly grated wasabi (or from a tube)
Reduced-sodium soy sauce, to use at the table

1. Place the eggs in a large bowl and whisk until just mixed.
2. In a small bowl, whisk together the dashi, sake, sugar, soy, and a generous pinch of salt until the sugar has dissolved. Add to the eggs and stir to combine. Transfer the egg mixture to a large glass measuring cup.
3. Place a medium nonstick rectangular-shaped skillet over medium heat. (If you do not have a rectangular skillet, you can use a round one.) Add 1/2 teaspoon of the oil and brush it over the surface of the skillet with a pastry brush. Working in batches, pour one eighth of the egg mixture into the skillet. Tilt the pan to coat the surface evenly with the egg. When the egg begins to pucker around the edges, push-roll the egg with chopsticks or a spatula (as if you were rolling a tortilla) toward the far end of the pan so that you have a long cylinder of egg. Keep the roll in the pan; you are going to use it to keep building a layered, log-shaped omelette.
4. With your first egg cylinder still sitting at one end of your skillet, add another 1/2 teaspoon of oil to the pan and brush it over the surface. Next, pour another eighth portion of the egg mixture into the skillet. Tip the pan slightly to make sure the skillet surface is evenly covered with egg, then gently lift up the cylinder of cooked egg to make sure the uncooked egg flows underneath it (this will make it easier to create your roll). This time, use the cooked egg cylinder as your core and roll it toward the handle side of the skillet so that the freshly cooked

egg rolls around the original egg cylinder. You should now have a slightly fatter cylinder of egg.

5. Continue cooking the remaining six portions of raw egg mixture in this manner, rolling the cylinder back and forth, brushing the skillet with ½ teaspoon of oil for each new batch, and using the expanding cylinder of egg as your core each time you roll. You may need to lower the heat when cooking the last batch to prevent the large roll from becoming too brown on the outside.

6. Transfer the egg log to a cutting board and slice it into 8 equal pieces. The easiest way to do this is to first cut the log in half, then cut each half in half again. Finally, cut the 4 pieces in half to yield 8 equal pieces.

7. Lay out 4 small serving plates and place 2 omelette pieces, cut side up to show the layers, in the center of each plate. Arrange the grated daikon in a mound on a small plate, along with the wasabi. Bring to the table and let diners season their omelettes with the daikon, wasabi, and soy as desired.

THE SIXTH PILLAR: TEA

You are walking down a garden path of sculpted stepping-stones.

Shafts of sunlight shimmer through the leaves of a towering ginkgo tree and settle on the dew-streaked moss.

Rounding a curve in the path, you see before you the teahouse, a thatch-roofed, multichambered hut made of bamboo and timber. It looks so rustic it could have sprung up directly from the forest floor.

You remove your shoes, step through a small door, and enter the floating world of tranquility and contemplation known as "*chanoyu*," or the Japanese tea ceremony.

Your kimono-clad hostess bows warmly and beckons you into a room of striking simplicity. Four straw tatami mats cover the floor. A single white camellia flower blossom rests in a bamboo vase, carefully placed to lean in your direction. Water in an iron urn is simmering over a charcoal fire. The room has no furniture and nothing else in it except various implements related to the serving of tea.

There is no beverage more Japanese than green tea, and the

ritual you are about to witness, rooted in Zen Buddhism and evolved slowly over five centuries, is a spiritual celebration of tea. "The tea ceremony requires years of training and practice," wrote the nineteenth-century journalist Lafcadio Hearn, "yet the whole of this art, as to its detail, signifies no more than the making and serving of a cup of tea. The supremely important matter is that the act be performed in the most perfect, most polite, most graceful, most charming manner possible."

The movements unfold like a classical ballet. Following a precise sequence of steps, the hostess cleans and displays the utensils to you: a carved bamboo tea scoop, a ceramic tea bowl. You are offered a small sweet to cleanse your palate.

When the kettle makes the whistling sound that Japanese call "the wind in the pines," it is removed and allowed to cool a bit as the hostess scoops green tea powder, or matcha, into the tea bowl. Like most tea, green tea comes from the evergreen camellia sinensis plant, but it is less processed than black teas, the leaves having been exposed to the process of oxidation for a shorter period of time. The tea used for matcha is especially unprocessed, young and fresh.

Adding water, your hostess whisks the mixture into a foamy broth and offers it to you.

The emotional heart of the tea ceremony, and of green tea, is the idea of treasuring a single moment in time. "In my own hands I hold a bowl of tea," wrote Soshitsu Sen XV, a twentieth-century grand master of the Urasenke tea sect. "I see all of nature represented in its green color. Closing my eyes, I find green mountains and pure water within my own heart. Silently, sitting alone, drinking tea, I feel these become part of me. Sharing this bowl of tea with others, they, too, become one with it and nature."

It is safe to say that Japanese people have been consumed with tea, especially green tea, for many centuries. A Zen monk named Eisai brought tea seeds to Japan from China in the late twelfth century, and in the Middle Ages, elite Japanese were holding tea-tasting parties where up to one hundred different varieties were sampled. Soon the masses were hooked too. Eventually, tea was even mixed with food in some dishes, as it still is today. In the country, for example, my grandmother made tea rice porridge, using tea plants the family grew on nearby hillsides in the nearly semitropical climate of Mie Prefecture.

American food writer Victoria Abbott Riccardi spent a year studying cuisine in Japan, where she discovered the summertime pleasures of introducing what she describes as the "bewitching herbal flavor" of green tea into desserts. "When the weather turns warm in Kyoto," she wrote in the *Washington Post,* "teahouses offer numerous matcha-flavored confections to enjoy: shaved ice drizzled with clear green tea syrup; spirals of sponge cake filled with fluffy matcha mousse; and matcha ice cream topped with fresh fruit and whipped cream."

The bonds between tea and food were forged in the rise of

Boil water, infuse tea, and drink.
That is all you need to know.

—Sen no Rikyu, sixteenth-century tea master

kaiseki ryori, the cuisine served in conjunction with the tea ceremony. On the night of September 21, 1590, for example, according to a written record of the event, the most influential tea master in history, Sen no Rikyu, invited four guests to his home in Kyoto for tea and dinner. It was a typical party at the tea guru's house, with each dish selected and timed to enhance the expectation and enjoyment of the tea. The first course was soup with vegetables and sea bream marinated with sake, accompanied by a bowl of rice. After a few refreshing belts of sake, out came servings of silken tofu, as well as broiled salmon. The party finished off with helpings of chestnuts and sweet soybean cakes. Then came the tea.

In my mother's Tokyo kitchen, hot green tea is a perpetual favorite. Every dinner finishes off with a small cup or two of freshly brewed sencha, the most popular grade of green tea in Japan. During the week she might also serve hojicha, a roasted green tea with a woodsy flavor, or English tea. On special occasions, she brings out the "king of the green teas": gyokuro, which is expensive, mellow-tasting, and slightly sweet.

In early summer she serves shin cha, which are young leaves made from the first harvest of the year. The drying process of the newly harvested tea leaves is much shorter than that of sencha, so shin cha has a fresh green flavor and aroma. Japanese people look forward to shin cha's arrival every year and enjoy it during May and June, when it is *shun* (in season).

I like the straight-and-pure grassy taste of sencha any time of the day. I also like genmaicha, a mixture of lesser quality green tea and roasted brown rice. And I love genmaimatcha, a mixture of genmaicha and matcha, the powdered green tea used for tea ceremonies. It is a study in contrasts—matcha's bitterness with the rice grain's earthy sweetness; and the powdered texture with bits of the grains.

To me, the intensely pure, clean, and brisk taste of green tea conjures up a range of emotions: relaxation, quiet rejuvenation, the joy of life, the feeling of springtime and early summer.

Japanese people have long connected drinking tea with health and longevity. The Zen monk Eisai, founder of Japan's tea craze, published a book in 1211 called *Drink Tea and Prolong Life*. In it, he called tea the "elixir that creates the mountain-dwelling immortal." He asserted that "tea is the most wonderful medicine for preserving health; it is the secret of long life. It shoots forth its leaves on the hillside like the spirit of the earth."

Later the health-giving aspects of green tea came to the attention of the West too. In the 1690s, a young Dutch doctor-in-training named Engelbert Kaempfer made a grand tour of Japan, and he could barely contain his enthusiasm for Japanese tea. "I believe that there is no Plant as yet known in the world," he gushed in his travel journal, "whose infusion or decoction, taken so very plentifully, as that of Tea in Japan, sits so easy upon the stomach, passes quicker through the body, or so gently refreshes the dropping animal spirits, and recreates the mind."

Kaempfer went on to offer an analysis of the medical benefits: "To sum up the virtues of this liquor in a few words, it opens the obstructions, cleanses the blood, and more particularly washes away that tartarous matter, which is the cause of calculous concretions, nephritick and goudy distempers."

I have no idea what he's talking about, but—who knows?—if we were to translate this into modern medicalese, perhaps he might have a point.

More recently, green tea has been the recipient of a tidal wave of positive press, based on various medical studies that spotlight its antioxidant and disease-fighting potential. Green tea has been touted as a cancer fighter, a cholesterol lowerer, a heart protector, and a fat burner. It can supposedly lower blood pressure, fight diabetes, delay Alzheimer's disease, and even help fight allergies.

One big green tea fan is Dr. Andrew Weil, clinical professor of internal medicine at the University of Arizona in Tucson. In his book *Eating Well for Optimum Health,* he cites a specific antioxidant in green tea, known as EGCG, as showing "impressive activity against many kinds of cancer" while appearing to protect the heart and arteries from oxidative damage.

The science on green tea is encouraging, but not conclusive, according to some experts. "We have thousands of years of history with green tea, and very little clinical research," says Dr. Frank L. Meyckens Jr., director of the cancer center at the University of California–Irvine. "We haven't proven how it works—or if it works." The trouble with many of the claims being made for green tea is that they are not based on the scientific gold standard of research—controlled, randomized clinical trials conducted on humans.

In July 2005, the Food and Drug Administration rejected a proposal to label green tea as a cancer fighter, ruling that "no credible evidence" currently supported the claim. The bottom line on green tea, concludes Professor Jeffrey Blumberg, a nutrition and antioxidants researcher at Tufts University, is that "it's a noncaloric beverage. It tastes good. It may even contain things that are beneficial. Two cups of green tea contain about as many flavonoids [a type of antioxidant] as a serving of fruit or vegetables. It's a potentially healthy choice the consumer can make when selecting a beverage." But, he noted, "tea is not a magic bullet for preventing cancer or heart disease."

For me, all talk of antioxidants and other disease-fighting ingredients aside, one of the main advantages of green tea is that it has about half the caffeine of coffee, making for a much mellower experience. And since I have cold green tea or mugicha (barley tea) so often, I'm completely bypassing the temptation to drink sodas, which means I avoid massive amounts of sugar, or the chemical sweeteners that are used in diet soft drinks. In fact, Billy and I keep a pitcher of naturally caffeine- and sugar-free mugicha in our refrigerator all the time, and drink it with breakfast, dinner, and any time between meals when we feel thirsty.

The other main advantage of tea—especially green tea—is, quite simply, that I love it. And now, after all this talk of tea, I am getting thirsty for a cup of sencha. I think I'll brew some green tea as a late-day lift-me-up for Billy and me.

Meanwhile, let us have a sip of tea. The afternoon glow is brightening the bamboos, the fountains are bubbling with delight, the soughing of the pines is heard in our kettle. Let us dream of evanescence, and linger in the beautiful foolishness of things.

—Kakuzo Okakura, The Book of Tea

Brewing Japanese Teas

SERVES 4

Sencha

4 teaspoons of loose tea leaves
2 cups of hot but not boiling water (about 175°F—or bring
the water to a boil and let it sit for 5 minutes before
pouring)
Steeping Time: 1 to 1½ minutes

Gyokuro

7 teaspoons of loose tea leaves
2 cups of hot but not boiling water (about 140°F—or
bring the water to a boil and let it sit for 20 minutes
before pouring)
Steeping Time: 2½ minutes

Hojicha, Genmaicha, or Genmaimatcha

3 teaspoons of loose tea leaves
2 cups of boiling water
Steeping Time: 30 seconds

1. Place the green tea leaves in a teapot.
2. Pour the hot water (at the temperature appropriate to the type
you are serving) and let the leaves steep for the time specified

above. Since different varieties of tea require amounts, water temperatures, and steeping times that may vary slightly from my directions, please follow the directions on the package if they differ from mine.

3. Lay out 4 teacups. Fill each cup one eighth full, then make the round of the 4 cups again, filling them another eighth of the way. Repeat until you have used the very last drop of the brewed green tea. The point of doing this is to ensure that you are serving the same strength of tea to all your guests. The teacups should be filled halfway or two thirds of the way to the rim. Do not leave any liquid in the teapot because the tea becomes bitter when it cools.

4. You can reuse the same leaves for a second serving. Simply repeat steps 2 and 3 when you are ready to serve the next round of tea.

Cold Mugicha (Barley Tea)

Pop 1 mugicha tea bag in a quart of cold water and let the mixture steep overnight in the refrigerator. The next morning your mugicha will be ready. (Each mugicha brand may require a different amount of water and steeping time. Please read the directions on the package.)

THE SEVENTH PILLAR: FRUIT

One day in 1878, a woman on horseback in the Japanese countryside chanced upon a sight that filled her with awe.

An Englishwoman, her name was Isabella Bird and she was
wandering the backwoods districts north of Tokyo in a time
when samurai still lived. "It was a lovely summer day, though
very hot," she remembered, "and the snowy peaks of Aidzu
scarcely looked cool as they glittered in the sunlight."

Then she came upon the plain of Yonezawa, and a vision of
a natural paradise so powerful that she called it "a perfect garden of Eden"—"an Asiatic Arcadia." She was stunned at the
"rich profusion" of fruit, vegetables, and herbs spread out before her in the sunny fields: melons, persimmons, apricots,
pomegranates, figs, rice, beans, cucumbers, eggplant, walnuts,
hemp, and indigo.

"It is an enchanting region of beauty, industry and comfort,
mountain girdled, and watered by the bright Matsuka
[River]," she recalled in her 1880 book *Unbeaten Tracks in
Japan*. "Everywhere there are prosperous and beautiful farm-

ing villages, with large houses with carved beams and ponderous tiled roofs, each standing in its own grounds, buried among persimmons and pomegranates, with flower-gardens under trellised vines, and privacy secured by high, closely-clipped screens of pomegranate and cryptomeria."

The land itself, thought Isabella Bird, seemed to smile.

When I think of Isabella's vision, I have to smile too, because it reminds me of my own "fruit heaven" at my father's childhood home in Kozaka in Mie Prefecture. The farm he grew up on was deep in the mountains, ensconced between two large rivers, the Kushida and the Miya, with abundant rain and warm gentle weather. It was a perfect place to grow fruit. Three types of tangerines flourished in the area, as did many other kinds of fruits, and vegetables too.

The plump, juicy tangerines (known as mikan, similar to mandarin oranges) grew in the family's hillside orchard and were the prize product of the farm. A small warehouse kept them cool after harvesting, ensuring that they would get to market almost as fresh as when they were picked, and with all of their nutrients intact. Those tangerines were treated with great care, for not only were they packed with goodies like vitamin A, vitamin C, and fiber, they were also like money in the bank.

The family fruit business was a low-tech, high-touch operation. At night my father and his brothers would help their father, Kumezo, polish baskets full of tangerines to a shiny orange glow and load them onto a wheeled cart.

Before 5 A.M. the next day, they'd set off with the cart and an escort bicycle, pushing and pulling the fruit-laden cart, on foot, through the surrounding hills and valleys, a full seven miles to the fruit and vegetable market in the city of Matsusaka. They also made side trips for deliveries to regular customers in villages along the way. After a long day of fruit wheeling and dealing, Kumezo would treat the boys to bowls of udon at a noodle shop.

When I visited the farm in summer as a little girl, I remember peeking into the warehouse and staring, awestruck, at the mountains of tangerines ripening on the shelves.

I felt like Alice in a Wonderland of Orange.

Both at home and at my grandparents' farm, fruit was our usual dessert. In Japan, a typical home-cooked meal ends not with a piece of cake or pie, or bowlsful of ice cream—but with tea and small cut-up pieces of fresh fruit.

Sometimes fruit will be replaced by a small plate of sweets—assorted cookies, or little sweet bean pastries—or green tea ice cream, but they will be bite-size compared with Western portions. Due to the traditionally small (or nonexistent) ovens in Japan, we haven't developed much of a baked dessert tradition in home cooking.

My father never had any cakes, pies, or cookies when he was growing up. Instead, he and his siblings went to the nearby hillsides and picked fruit and nuts—persimmons, strawberries, and chestnuts—for their snacks and desserts.

Statistically speaking, Japanese people don't eat more fruit per capita than people in the West, but I think they are eating it fresher, in its more unprocessed forms, and more often as the main dessert course. They use fruit in other parts of the meal too, as my mother likes to do. Sometimes she puts sliced apples in curry so that the sweetness of the apple will play against the hot spicy flavor of the curry. She also likes to put finely chopped apples in salad dressings. Among her favorites for desserts are cherries, watermelons, grapes, persimmons, strawberries, and, naturally, tangerines, which my dad's family still send to my parents in Tokyo from the country.

Other popular fruits in Japan are Fuji apples (considered by some to be among the world's best), Japanese persimmon (*kaki*), Japanese apricots (*ume*), pears (*nashi*), grapes, and melons. The highly aromatic rind of the yuzu fruit is used as a concentrated citrus flavoring in Japan, and is increasingly popular in fine restaurants in Europe and the United States.

What might the Japanese approach to dessert have to do with health and longevity?

For one thing, by eating fruit instead of large amounts of cookies, cakes, donuts, pies, and other baked goods (especially the packaged versions of those foods), the Japanese are avoiding one of the main sources of trans fats, which are under increasing attack by nutrition experts for their role in promoting cardiovascular disease. Other sources of trans fats include packaged chips, crackers, and muffins, as well as a lot of the fried and baked foods sold in fast food restaurants.

Over a decade ago, Dr. Walter Willett, chairman of Harvard University's School of Public Health nutrition department, wrote: "It can be conservatively estimated that approximately 30,000 deaths per year in the U.S. are attributable to trans fatty acids from partially hydrogenated vegetable oil."

As Professor Barry Popkin of the University of North Carolina explained on National Public Radio in 2003, "This trans-fatty acid molecule has very important effects on us in terms of cardiovascular disease and cancers. It's been shown to be much more dangerous than, for example, the saturated fat. So recently, the National Academy of Science and Institute of Medicine essentially said we should eat very little of it, if any." Professor David Katz of the Yale University School of Medicine calls trans fats "very clearly harmful to health, and not necessary."

In August 2005, the health department of New York City asked that all restaurants voluntarily stop using trans fats in food preparations. No one has made them illegal yet, but given how harmful trans fats are, perhaps they should be.

On the plus side of the equation, fruit consumption is a key component of the diets most commonly endorsed by leading doctors, scientists, and nutritional experts and researchers around the world, such as the Mediterranean diet, the Asian diet, and the DASH (Dietary Approaches to Stop Hypertension) diet.

Comparing the Mediterranean and Japanese diets, Dr. Antonia Trichopoulou, professor of medicine at the University of Athens, notes, "the common denominators point to a beneficial role of fruits, vegetables and legumes, not to mention the low energy intake and high fish consumption which characterizes the Japanese diet."

"The Japanese diet is a very good one, perhaps the best," says cardiologist Dr. Robert Vogel of the University of Maryland. "Their diet is substantially fruit/vegetable/complex carbohydrate based, whereas ours is animal/simple sugar based."

Dr. Dean Ornish, the leading diet authority who was recently hired as a nutritional consultant by none other than McDonald's, gave fruit a boost when he recommended in a recent issue of *Time*: "Eat more 'good carbs' like fruits, vegetables, legumes and unrefined grains such as whole-wheat flour and brown rice. They are rich in fiber, which slows absorption and fills you up before you take in too many calories."

And fruit is one of the stars of the 2005 U.S. Dietary Guidelines issued by the federal government, which urge us to "increase your daily intake of fresh fruits and vegetables, and whole grains." Among the benefits cited by the guidelines are their high fiber content, and the fact that most fruits are relatively low in calories. The guidelines also endorse fruits as "important sources of at least eight additional nutrients, including vitamin C, folate, and potassium (which may help control blood pressure)."

Greater consumption of both fruits and vegetables, according to the guidelines, is associated with a reduced risk of stroke and perhaps other cardiovascular diseases, and a reduced risk of certain cancers, such as oral cavity and pharynx, larynx, lung, esophagus, stomach, and colon-rectum. "Moreover, increased consumption of fruits and vegetables may be a useful component of programs designed to achieve and sustain weight loss."

I'll tell you the secret of serving fruit in my mother's Tokyo kitchen: it is all in the presentation. Fruits are peeled, sliced into mini-masterpieces of natural beauty, and arranged on small pretty plates of stoneware or earthenware or china.

When I was growing up, my mother was always conscious of the visual appeal of the food she put on the table. But now she is studying the art of Thai-style food carving and has taken that interest to a whole new level. On my last visit to

Japan, she showed me over fifty fruit-carving designs she was working on using mock-ups of bars of soap. They looked like chrysanthemums and dahlias in varying sizes and colors.

Inspired by my mother, let me suggest that for your next dessert, instead of cake, a bowl of ice cream, or a plate of jumbo cookies, you try this:

- Select three types of fresh fruit in season.
- Slice and assemble them into shapes resembling flowers, stars, crescent moons, and other objects in nature or from your imagination.
- Arrange them elegantly on beautiful plates.
- Admire their beauty and savor the distinctive taste of each of the three fruits.

When you're finished enjoying your fruit masterpieces, congratulate yourself by saying, *"Gochiso-sama,"* which means, "That was a feast!"

You are now an artist—working in the medium of natural fruit.

Food should be eaten with the eyes as well as the mouth.
Serving food is like painting a picture.
Food should be arranged like exquisite jewelry.

—Chizuko Moriyama

TOKYO KITCHEN SAMPLE MEALS

Now that you have seen all of the recipes in this book, here are some ideas for how to put them together to create whole meals. A typical Japanese meal at home, especially dinner, consists of:

- A bowl of rice
- Miso or clear soup
- Three side dishes with a variety of ingredients

The dishes are served more or less at once, unlike a formal Western-style meal, or a multicourse meal at a fine Japanese restaurant, or kaiseki. With Japanese home-cooked meals, you eat a small amount from every dish and work your way around them, instead of focusing on only one dish at a time.

When a noodle dish is served, it replaces rice in the menu; typically soup is not served then, since noodle dishes come with a broth. When cooked ingredients are used as toppings for rice or noodles, like beef over rice, chicken and eggs over rice, or shrimp tempura over soba noodles, there may be only one or two small side dishes. A dish with a topping tends to be a casual, on-the-go, light meal, making it perfect for lunch.

Sample Breakfasts

Breakfast 1 is a typical traditional Japanese breakfast. Each portion is small, but it is a full, energy-packed meal.

BREAKFAST 1

Cooked Brown or White Rice

Miso Soup with Daikon and Tofu

A small piece of Pan-Fried Atlantic Mackerel

One or two slices of Tamago (Japanese Omelette)

Small pieces of nori sea vegetables (seaweed)

Green tea

Breakfast 2 is a variation on the preceding à la my mother's Tokyo kitchen. The soup is so hearty that you only need rice.

BREAKFAST 2

Cooked Brown or White Rice

Snap Peas, Daikon, and Egg Soup

Green tea

Breakfast 3 is a power breakfast, my way: rice, miso soup, mountain and sea vegetables, and egg in one.

BREAKFAST 3

Japanese Country Power Breakfast, sprinkled with shredded nori seaweed

Sample Lunches

Lunches tend to have fewer dishes than dinners, mostly because people are in a hurry!

LUNCH 1

Japanese Comfort Food: Rice Balls

Tokyo Salad

Green tea

LUNCH 2

Cold Soba Buckwheat Noodles

Tamago—Japanese-Style Omelette

Tasty Summer Edamame

Green tea

LUNCH 3

Chicken and Eggs over Rice

Miso Soup with Daikon and Tofu

Green tea

LUNCH 4

The Perfect Bowl of Soba Noodles

Kinpira—Burdock and Carrot

Green tea

Sample Dinners

When assembling a meal, especially dinner, I try to balance a variety of ingredients, flavors, textures, and cooking methods among the dishes. I'll match a fish dish with egg and vegetable dishes, chicken with two vegetable dishes, or three dishes made of different types of vegetables.

For a variety of flavors, I combine a sweet or spicy dish with a more subtly flavored dish. When combining, I think of the flavors derived not only from seasonings or garnishes, but from the main ingredients. I may combine the sweet fatty Teriyaki Fish with the vinegared Tokyo Salad, or bring the sweet Spinach with Sesame Seeds together with the dashi-simmered Hijiki Sea Vegetable and Tofu. Mixing textures means crunchy with soft, and liquid-filled with dry or solid. Combining various cooking methods brings simmered and fried together, and cooked and raw.

DINNER 1

Cooked Brown or White Rice

Miso Soup with Short-Neck Clams

Spinach with Sesame Seeds

Tokyo Fried Chicken

Hijiki Sea Vegetable and Fried Tofu

Green tea

Dessert: Sliced fresh fruit

DINNER 2

Cooked Brown or White Rice

Miso Soup with Daikon and Tofu

Salmon-Edamame Burger

Eggplant Sautéed with Miso

Chilled Tofu with Bonito Flakes and Chopped Scallions

Green tea

DINNER 3

Cooked Brown or White Rice

Clear Soup with Tofu and Shiitake Mushrooms

Teriyaki Fish

Mom's Carrot-Tofu Dish

Spinach with Bonito Flakes

Green tea

DINNER 4

Cooked Brown or White Rice

Naomi's Gyoza Dumplings

Tokyo Salad

Green tea

Dessert: Sliced fresh fruit

DINNER 5

Cooked Brown or White Rice

Miso Soup with Short-Neck Clams

Shrimp and Vegetable Tempura

Kiriboshi Daikon with Shiitake Mushrooms and Tofu

Simmered Succulent Tofu

Green tea

DINNER 6

Cooked Brown or White Rice

Clear Soup with Tofu and Shiitake Mushrooms

Smoked Salmon Rolls with Shiso and Kaiware

Stir-Fried Vegetables

Green tea

Dessert: Sliced fresh fruit

Ease-into-It Starter Selections:

To begin Japanese-style home cooking, I recommend these selections from the above meals to ease you into the swing of it. Breakfast is a great way to get started.

BREAKFAST 3

Japanese Country Power Breakfast, sprinkled with shredded nori seaweed

Then, when you feel ready to take a bigger bite of your new Tokyo kitchen, start incorporating more Japanese meals like these over a period of several days.

LUNCH 1

Japanese Comfort Food: Rice Balls

Tokyo Salad

Green tea

LUNCH 3

Chicken and Eggs over Rice

Miso Soup with Daikon and Tofu

Green tea

DINNER 1

Cooked Brown or White Rice

Miso Soup with Short-Neck Clams

Spinach with Sesame Seeds

Tokyo Fried Chicken

Hijiki Sea Vegetable and Fried Tofu

Green tea

Dessert: Sliced fresh fruit

CHAPTER 6

The Samurai Diet

The samurai swords, the costumes, the amazing landscapes.
There's just something about it all that is eternally cool.

—Tom Cruise

THE HISTORY OF JAPAN may have turned on a battle between brown rice and white rice.

It was a battle that unleashed one of the world's most powerful woman warriors.

Step into the time machine with me.
Let's fly backward, say 820 years or so. . . .

The greatest female samurai in the history of Japan was described as "especially beautiful, with white skin, long hair, and charming features." She loved horses—and she loved combat.

She rode at the head of 50,000 mounted troops and foot soldiers, beside her boyfriend and boss, a swashbuckling, wise-cracking, and dangerously unstable general named Yoshinaka Minamoto.

Her name was Tomoe Gozen.

Together, Tomoe Gozen and Yoshinaka Minamoto gal-loped into a lightning-fast string of stunning, bloody military triumphs. The summer of the year 1183 brought them to the outskirts of the ancient capital of Kyoto, and to a turning point in history, the impact of which the Japanese would feel for the next seven hundred years.

And according to one theory, as Tomoe Gozen, her general, and their forces gathered in the hills in their torchlit camps for the final strike toward the prize of the capital city, they had a se-cret weapon. It was wrapped up in their packs and in their pockets, and it gave them a crucial edge in energy, stamina, and battlefield performance over the enemy armies arrayed against them.

The secret weapon was brown rice.

———

Tomoe Gozen was among the rarest of historical figures, a woman samurai, and she traveled in a twilight world between myth and history, where fact and legend are impossible to sep-arate. She may have been a literary device, or she may have been a flesh-and-blood woman. But the medieval literary clas-sic *The Tale of the Heike* portrays her as one of the most skilled and ferocious warriors the world had ever seen.

"She was also a remarkably strong archer," the story went, "and as a swordswoman she was a warrior worth a thousand, ready to confront a demon or a god, mounted or on foot. She handled unbroken horses with superb skill; she rode unscathed down perilous descents. Whenever a battle was imminent, Yoshinaka sent her out as his first captain, equipped with strong armor, an oversized sword, and a mighty bow; and she performed more deeds of valor than any of his other warriors."

Tomoe Gozen and her lover came from one of Japan's most beautiful and isolated places, a region now called Nagano, in the heart of the Japanese Alps. It is a land of pine forests, crashing waterfalls, boiling hot springs, and 9,000-foot gossamer peaks, where wild vegetables and chestnut trees blossom among alpine flowers on verdant hillsides.

Their army charged down from the mountains at the vanguard of a revolution led by a great samurai clan, the Minamotos, who were devoted to overthrowing the rival Taira clan, who held the capital, the emperor, and half the country in the grip of a corrupt court bureaucracy. It was a chaotic, complex, and hyperviolent blood feud.

The man Tomoe Gozen was in love with, her commander-in-chief Yoshinaka Minamoto, was gifted at dazzling strategy on the battlefield and given to cocky, poetic outbursts about his triumphs there. "I fought them again and again," he boasted as the final battle with the enemy loomed. "I devised stratagems in camp; I won victories on the field. Whenever I struck, the foe yielded; whenever I attacked, the enemy capitulated. It was not different from an autumn wind ravaging plantain leaves; it was the same as a winter frost withering trees and grasses."

This was full-scale civil war, a struggle as epic as the Trojan

War. And the combatants, in a provocative theory put forward by the twenty-first-century Japanese food historian Hisao Nagayama, were engaged in what was ultimately a clash between "soft-rice eaters" and "hard-rice eaters."

The Taira clan, Nagayama believes, had grown soft and lazy whiling away the years in the luxuriant capital city, extorting taxes from the peasants of the countryside, busying themselves with poetry, music, and flower arrangement—and eating tender foods and white rice.

The warriors of the country-dwelling Minamoto clan, by contrast, grew strong and fierce on their diet of brown rice, fish, and pickled vegetables, a diet that sharpened their minds and fighting spirits.

When Tomoe Gozen and the Minamoto forces entered Kyoto in triumph, the petrified enemy had already fled the capital in terror, and at first, the occupiers were hailed as saviors.

It was absolute victory—for wholesome brown rice.

Nagayama's theory, unusual as it might seem, is not impossible to believe, since food can have a decisive influence on history. In fact, the economy and politics of Japan during the Heian era (794–1185) are often linked to rice, as a tax payment and as a source of national crisis during droughts and famines.

But then, with the people's applause still ringing in his ears, Tomoe Gozen's beloved general Yoshinaka Minamoto managed to make a mess of things almost immediately. Though he was a great warrior, he was a spectacularly incompetent administrator.

First, he started dallying with an unknown number of local women, to the annoyance of his troops (and presumably of Tomoe Gozen). Much worse, from a historical perspective, he allowed his soldiers to go on a weeks-long rampage of partying, looting, and pillaging that horrified the elegant residents of Kyoto, leading to clashes across the city, lots of heads being cut off, and the incineration of the palace in a great fire.

As things fell apart, the general dithered in fantasies. "Should I become Emperor?" he mused (in a passage from *The Tale of the Heike*). "I rather like the idea of being Emperor, but it would not do for me to adopt a boy's hairstyle."

Within weeks it all collapsed into a family feud worthy of Shakespeare—or *The Sopranos*.

The ultimate boss of the Minamoto family, a warlord named Yoritomo Minamoto, was outraged at his cousin Yoshinaka's tragic fumbling of the great prize, and he sent 60,000 troops from the east to chase him out of the capital and kill him.

Through all this mess, the fearless Tomoe Gozen stuck by her man. She and Yoshinaka fled with their last remaining 300 mounted samurai (down from the original 50,000). But they were trapped by an advance force of 6,000 fellow Minamoto warriors not far from Kyoto, and chose to make a last stand.

In classic samurai-on-the-edge fashion, Yoshinaka stood tall in his stirrups, screamed boasts at the enemy, and gave the order to charge. The outnumbered band was nearly cut to pieces, but Tomoe Gozen and her lover somehow punched their way through in hand-to-hand combat and broke free, their small band of warriors now down to 50. And soon, after zigzagging and slashing through several more layers of enemy fighters, only 5 of Yoshinaka's troops were left alive.

Now the vain Yoshinaka, who liked to be called Lord Kiso (after the Kiso Valley, near his hometown), ordered Tomoe Gozen to flee, not for her own safety, but to spare him personal embarrassment. "Quickly, now," he commanded. "You are a woman, so be off with you, go wherever you please. I intend to die in battle, or to kill myself if I am wounded. It would be unseemly to let people say, 'Lord Kiso kept a woman with him during his last battle.'"

At first she obeyed, and began riding off the battlefield.

Then, according to *The Tale of the Heike,* she pulled up her reins, deciding, "If only I could find a worthy foe! I would fight a last battle for His Lordship to watch."

At this, she allegedly charged into a team of 30 opposing samurai, twisted off their leader's head, hurled it to the ground, and managed to escape. Her boyfriend was quickly hunted down in the woods, where he committed suicide by diving from his horse onto a sword.

At last report, Tomoe Gozen threw away her helmet and armor and vanished toward the eastern provinces, never to be heard from again. One story has her becoming a nun and living until age ninety.

On the larger scale of history, though, Tomoe Gozen's struggle and that of the brown-rice-loving Minamoto clan was hardly in vain. The momentum established by the capture of Kyoto was seized upon by boss Yoritomo Minamoto's forces, who chased the doomed Taira armies across Japan until they were able to throw them—literally—into the ocean in a final climactic sea battle at Dannoura in April 1185.

Yoritomo Minamoto eventually declared himself shogun, or military ruler, of all Japan. Suddenly the samurai, and not the royal aristocracy, were the rulers of Japan—as they would be for the next seven centuries. The samurai were now Japan's full-time elite warrior class.

The institutions of government established by Yoritomo, the first shogun and the winner of what we might call the "Brown Rice vs. White Rice War," would last from 1185 until the collapse of the shogunate and the twilight of the samurai in 1868.

———

The eating habits of the victorious Minamoto family and their successors illustrate an intriguing point: the "samurai diet," in many of its key elements, represents one of the purest forms of Japanese traditional cuisine.

"Even when the shogunate was well established," wrote historian Stephen Turnbull in his *Samurai: The Story of Japan's Great Warriors*, "it was still unusual to see samurai eating polished [white] rice except on feast days." The samurai, according to Turnbull, lived largely on brown rice mixed with wheat or millet, plus fruit and vegetables like eggplant, cucumbers, and mushrooms. "If they lived near the sea there was the addition of fish, shellfish and seaweed," he wrote. "River fish and game were also available, and samurai were enthusiastic hunters."

Throughout the nearly 700-year reign of the samurai, through civil wars and foreign wars, periods of anarchy, and periods of stability and great cultural flourishing, the outlines of the samurai diet remained constant, sometimes supplemented by dishes of poultry or wild boar—the latter cleverly named "mountain whale" to skirt the prohibition against eating land animals.

The samurai diet helped fuel a permanent class of millions

of warriors. A few of these warriors were chivalrous, some were pure killers, and most of them were in business strictly for themselves. "They were a kind of mafiosi," wrote samurai scholar Mitsuo Kure, "who fought for family, land and plunder, but scarcely for honor."

In action, they were the ultimate alpha males, some of them as fierce as Tomoe Gozen. They talked tough. They fought tough. They ate tough, scrounging food off the land, chewing wild nuts, and cooking brown rice in their battle helmets.

They even wrote tough. One samurai from the twelfth century recorded in his diary: "I spurred my horse on frowning precipices, careless of death in the face of the foe. I braved the dangers of wind and wave, not reckoning that my body might sink to the bottom of the sea, and be devoured by monsters of the deep. My pillow was my harness, arms my trade."

The samurai did manage to hold Japan together more or less, and as the years passed they became tea ceremony enthusiasts, art collectors—and notorious fashionistas.

Over time, the samurai also became food connoisseurs. A scroll painting from the Kamakura period (1185–1333) shows a seated group of armored warriors eating heaping bowls of rice from individual tables, along with several little side dishes each, with a cup of sake. A typical samurai family wedding in the 1400s might feature a dish like yams and pheasant cutlets simmered in miso, garnished with sprinkled seaweed. In the Edo period (1603–1868), samurai traveled to the imperial court carrying New Year's gifts of salted salmon.

For many samurai, Tokyo (then called Edo) was gourmet food mecca.

One country samurai from the Tanabe clan named Harada

loved the food in the capital so much that he wrote a guide-book for other samurai called *The Pride of Edo*, singing the praises of noodle shops and sweet buns. Harada's guidebook appeared in the mid-1800s.

The eating habits of the samurai of the twelfth through eighteenth centuries seem very close to what we now think of as the traditional Japanese diet—and are not too far from the recommendations of many twenty-first-century doctors, scientists, and nutritionists.

Dr. Laurence Sperling, director of preventive cardiology at the Emory University School of Medicine in Atlanta, notes that "the traditional Japanese diet is very similar to the three dietary approaches that appear to be the healthiest, sustainable long-term approaches—the Mediterranean, DASH [Dietary Approaches to Stop Hypertension], and hunter-gatherer diets." And, according to Professor Marion Nestle, chair of the Department of Nutrition and Food Studies at New York University, "The Asian diet meets every recommendation you can think of for what you need to help chronic diseases. Infinitely varied and delicious, it's a nutritionist's dream."

However, it has to be admitted that a few hundred years ago, the Japanese took a slight wrong turn from their historically ultrahealthy eating habits—by taking a detour into white rice exclusively.

For some reason, brown rice fell out of favor in Japan. White rice became the standard table rice, and it remains so today, even though experts believe brown rice is more nutritious. This may be changing, as a small but growing number of health-conscious Japanese women are beginning to experiment with, and switch over to, brown rice. Brown rice products are popping up in Tokyo convenience stores, too, and some brown-rice-friendly restaurants have recently been spotted.

THE BROWN RICE CHALLENGE

One Way to Ride the Whole Grains Trend

The 2005 U.S. Dietary Guidelines urge us to *eat more whole grains*, including this direct challenge to eat brown rice: "To eat more whole grains, substitute a whole-grain product for a refined product—such as eating whole-wheat bread instead of white bread or brown rice instead of white rice. For a change, try brown rice or whole-wheat pasta."

. Here's one way to do it: for a period of two weeks, eat servings of brown rice instead of less nutritious choices like white bread, rolls, or trans-fat-heavy muffins or cookies. Or include brown rice at breakfast instead of non-whole-grain pancakes or waffles. Then, at the end of two weeks, ask yourself how much better you feel.

I love white rice, and it's clearly a lot healthier than lots of other foods. But I love brown rice just as much—it's nutty, complex, savory, and satisfying—and it's even healthier than white rice. A bowl of brown rice is a perfect complement to almost any dish.

THE SAMURAI SHOPPING LIST

How to Eat Like a Warrior

If you and your husband, wife, or partner are ready to unleash your inner Tomoe Gozen and Tom-Cruise-in-a-kimono, here are some of the favorite samurai-type foods, most of which you can pick up at your neighborhood supermarket:

- Salmon
- Fresh vegetables, raw or lightly simmered
- Brown rice
- Miso soup (try low-sodium)
- Tofu and soybeans
- Fresh fruit
- Green tea
- Chestnuts (called victory chestnuts, they were eaten by samurai before a battle for good luck)

12 EASY TOKYO TIPS

How to Start Living Like a Healthy Japanese Woman Today

To summarize the lessons of Japanese food history—and my mother's Tokyo kitchen:

1. Practice *hara hachi bunme*—eat until you are 80 percent full.
2. Become a master portion controller—serve modest-size portions on small, beautiful tableware.

3. Eat and chew your food at a leisurely pace, savoring every bite.

4. Take special time to admire the beauty of your food and its presentation.

5. Eat more fish, fresh fruit, and vegetables—and fewer saturated fats and trans fats.

6. Cook with canola oil or rice bran oil.

7. Treat yourself to a Japanese power breakfast: miso soup with vegetables, egg, and tofu.

8. Think of vegetables more often as a main dish—and red meat as a side or occasional dish.

9. Have a bowl of short-grain white or brown rice with your meals instead of white bread, muffins, or rolls.

10. Instead of sweetened soda, drink cold unsweetened Japanese tea.

11. Walk everywhere you can.

12. Remember that loving to eat well is an important part of being healthy—and that cooking and eating should be fun.

• Bonus tip for living even healthier: eat less sodium and more whole grains.

The Great Food Offering

It will happen, perhaps, one day in the not-too-distant future.

A Japanese woman wearing a crown with a black plume and white ceremonial robes will walk slowly down a wooded path toward a sacred shrine, at the head of a torchlit procession of priests and attendants bearing ceremonial baskets of purified fish, rice, and fruit.

A thousand dignitaries in formal attire will be watching nearby, but the only sounds to be heard will be the crunching of heavy lacquered sandals upon pebbles and the strains of a Japanese flute echoing through the trees.

In a secret ritual mostly unchanged for 1,300 years, the

robed woman and her attendants will disappear from sight into the inner courtyards of the imperial palace in Tokyo, where she will begin the Great Food Offering Ceremony, or Daijosai, the final step in becoming the monarch of Japan, the incarnation of the oldest surviving royal family on earth.

Japan has had empresses before, as recently as the eighteenth century. After World War II, the Japanese legislature banned women from the throne, but it would take only a new law to be passed to allow a female heir apparent like the current little Princess Aiko (born in 2001) to become empress in the future.

The Japanese woman in her ceremonial robes and crown will enter a chamber that, according to legend, contains the living spirit of the sun goddess Amaterasu, the mythic founding mother of the Japanese nation, and the spirit credited with creating rice fields and rice cultivation.

The ritual will be almost identical to the ones performed by her father, and grandfather, and many of her ancestors before her, dating to the dawn of the Japanese monarchy.

Escorted now by just two female priests, it is believed that the empress will kneel down beside a rice straw bed that is said to contain the reclining spirit of the sun goddess.

The sun goddess and the empress will commune through the night, sharing thanksgiving offerings of rice and rice wine.

This ancient, eternally unchanging ceremony will be a vivid display of two of the forces that have nourished the Japanese soul since the moment of its creation:

The power of healthy food . . . and the power of women.

I am dreaming.

**I am submerged in thickly intertwined plots and
cinematic dream scenarios.**

Mixed with the voices and visions in the dreams, I begin to
hear faint noises far away. It's my husband, making breakfast.
In our house, Billy's in charge of breakfast. This is for two reasons—I can never wake up, and he makes a terrific Japanese-
style country breakfast.

I drag myself to the breakfast table, look out the window,
and admire the morning sunlight splashing the Chrysler and
Empire State buildings. Cars are honking on Second Avenue.

Breakfast appears. It is a steaming bowl of miso soup, brim-
ming with tofu and vegetables.

Most of the ingredients are from the local supermarket, but
some of the vegetables I grew myself—not here in New York,
where I don't have access to a garden, but in Westchester
County, where my mother-in-law, Marilou, lives.

This spring Marilou obtained a ten-by-twenty-foot plot in
her village community garden. I get up at the crack of dawn
every Saturday and take the train to Westchester to work in it
with her. So far, we've grown salad greens, tomatoes, cucumbers, mizuna, and twelve kinds of herbs from the farmers market, including basil, purple basil, thyme, and oregano. We're
also working on gooseberries, raspberries, chives, and mint.

Since I thought it would be great to grow some Japanese vegetables and herbs that are difficult to find in U.S. markets, I
googled their names and found the Kitazawa Seed Company in
California, which has been selling Japanese vegetable seeds since
1917. I went crazy and ordered a bunch of seed packets: negi,

kaiware, shungiku (chrysanthemum greens), komatsuna greens, shiso, and mitsuba (Japanese parsley). They even have hinona, a turnip that has greens which my grandmother used to make my favorite salad!

Thinking about my garden, I gaze at the bowl of soup and inhale the steamy aromas.

Bright red grape tomatoes and green beans are bobbing on the surface. The miso is making cloudy swirls around them.

I stir the soup and feel lots of chunky ingredients. I think I see some chopped potatoes, broccoli, and daikon.

I sip a spoonful. "Hmmmm." The rich flavor perks me up in a much gentler way than a sip of coffee.

The tomato tastes sweet. I scoop up a chunk of tofu. Billy has cut it into random abstract shapes. He claims it's a Frank Gehry–inspired composition.

"I love the tofu flavor and texture." I always say it no matter how many times I have this dish.

Then I find sections of the boiled egg that Billy sliced into the soup. The yolk is golden yellow and the middle portion is ever so slightly undercooked but not runny, just the way I like it. "Perfect! Look!" I show the egg yolk to Billy. He smiles as he stirs and sips his soup.

"How many minutes and seconds did you cook the eggs to make them so perfect?" I ask.

"I am not telling you," Billy replies. "It's the chef's secret for-mula."

"Wow, it tastes so good!" I marvel. I am now full of energy and ready to burst out the door and into the new day. This tastes so much like the miso soup my grandmother Tsune used to make for me.

Today, I'm not a hard-core 100 percent purist on the subject of Japanese food, by any means. I have cravings for thick juicy burgers and fries, and I act on them. Last Valentine's Day, Billy and I took the Q train to Di Fara's Pizzeria on Avenue J in Brooklyn, and devoured the greatest fully loaded fresh cheese pizza on Earth. Now and then I'll dig into a cup of Ben & Jerry's Chunky Monkey ice cream. I still drink more Starbucks than I do green tea.

But this way of eating, in the tradition of my family and in celebration of the natural beauty, flavor, and health of the earth's foods, is the way that makes me feel the happiest.

I plunge my spoon into the soup again and take in a big mouthful.

I think of some of the places I've been in my life and remember some of the great food I've tasted—in places like Paris, Rome, Portugal, Chicago, Kyoto, Hong Kong, New Orleans, San Francisco, London, Hawaii, and the Irish countryside.

Then it hits me.

And I am speechless. . . .

I am in the middle of New York City.

But I am also in a tangerine orchard in the Japanese countryside.

And I am in my mother's Tokyo kitchen.

Source Notes

Any quotations from experts that appear in the text but are not sourced below are from our telephone and e-mail interviews.

In addition to the books and articles cited, the publications *Food Culture* and *Food Forum,* published by Kikkoman Corporation, were a valuable source of historical background in researching this book, especially the essays of Japanese food scholar Zenjiro Watanabe. At the Special Collections Room at the Tokyo Metropolitan Central Library, we reviewed a variety of rare historical Japanese cookbooks dating back to the late 1600s.

Among the most valuable additional books we consulted are: Dennis Hirota, ed., *Wind in the Pines: Classic Writings of the Way of Tea as a Buddhist Path* (Fremont, Calif.: Asian Humanities Press, 1995); Yuko Fujita, *Recipes of Japanese Cooking* (Tokyo: Navi International, 2004); Emi Kazuko, *The Japanese Kitchen* (London: Southwater, 2002); Louis Frederic, *Daily Life in Japan at the Time of the Samurai,* trans. by Eileen M. Lowe (London: George Allen and Unwin, 1972); and Heihachi Tanaka with Betty Nicholas, *The Pleasures of Japanese Cooking* (Englewood Cliffs, N.J.: Prentice-Hall, 1963).

Introduction

1 Epigraph: *Lost in Translation*, written and directed by Sofia Coppola, distributed by Focus Features, 2003.

2 For the World Health Organization's data on the global obesity epidemic and its global spread, see "Obesity and Overweight Facts," on its Web site, http:www.who.int/ dietphysicalactivity/publications/fact/obesity/en/ (accessed August 2005).

2 "It's universal": Janie Magruder, "Arizona Looks for Solutions to Childhood Obesity," Associated Press Newswires, February 6, 2005.

3 For obesity rising among French, see Michael Fumento, "French Women Don't Get Fat? Wrong," *Deseret News* (Salt Lake City), March 27, 2005.

3 an estimated $117 billion: U.S. Department of Health and Human Services National Institutes of Health press release, "NIH Releases Research Strategy to Fight Obesity Epidemic," August 24, 2004, available at http://www.nih.gov/news/pr/ aug2004/niddk-24.htm. The comparable homeland security cost is from U.S. Congressional Budget Office Economic and Budget Issue Brief: "Federal Funding for Homeland Security: An Update," July 20, 2005, available at http://www.cbo.gov/ ftpdocs/65xx/doc6566/7-20-HomelandSecurity.pdf.

3 Dr. Julie Louise Gerberding: U.S. Centers for Disease Control and Prevention telebriefing transcript, "Overweight and Obesity: Clearing the Confusion," June 2, 2005, available at http://www.cdc.gov/od/oc/media/transcripts/t050602.htm.

3 "the obesity epidemic is more than a public health crisis . . .": California Department of Health Services news release, "Obesity Costs California $21.7 Billion Annually," April 5, 2005, available at http://www.dhs.ca.gov/ps/cdic/cpns/press/ downloads/CostofObesityPressRelease.pdf.

3 "It boggles my mind": Magruder, "Arizona Looks for Solutions to Childhood Obesity."

4 "I think epidemic's almost too polite . . .": Andrea Mayes, "Obese Children Turning to Surgery," *The Australian* (Sydney), May 13, 2005.

4 "counteract the increasing weight of passengers": Jessica Lawrence, "Excess Baggage: Bigger Planes Needed to Fit Oversized Passengers," *Sunday Mail* (Adelaide), November 21, 2004.

5 The table of obesity rates by country—and, unless otherwise noted, other obesity rates cited in this chapter—are from the International Obesity Task Force Web site, accessed August 2005. For full data and notes, see "Global Prevalence" in "Database" section of http://www.iotf.org.

5 "Japanese women set a new record . . .": Associated Press Newswires, July 16, 2004.

5 "the life expectancy of Japanese men and women . . .": "Japan: Healthcare and Pharmaceuticals Forecast," Economist Intelligence Unit, November 11, 2004.

5 Data for life expectancy at birth by country are from *World Health Organization World Health Report, 2005* (citing latest figures, as of 2003), available at http://www.who.int/whr/2005/annexes-en.pdf. Additionally, three "mini-states" enjoy high life expectancy at birth: Monaco (women: 85 years; men: 78 years; both sexes: 81 years) and Andorra and San Marino (for both: women: 84 years; men: 78 years; both sexes: 81 years).

5 Body Mass Index, or BMI, is a method of classifying overweight and obesity that factors in both weight and height. In adults, overweight is defined by the WHO as a BMI of >=25, and obesity is defined as a BMI of >=30. In Japan, obesity is often defined by health officials as a BMI of 25 and over, combining "overweight" and "obese" into a single category. Different national health authorities sometimes use different

BMI cut-offs to define overweight and obesity. The WHO, however, uses the definition of obesity as 30 BMI and above as a global baseline to compare different countries. In 2002, WHO experts found that "Asians generally have a higher percentage of body fat than white people of the same age, sex, and BMI. Also, the proportion of Asian people with risk factors for type-2 diabetes and cardiovascular disease is substantial even below the existing WHO BMI cut-off point [for overweight]" of 25 BMI. But the experts noted that lowering the cut-off values by three units, to adjust for risk differences, "as seems appropriate for Hong Kong Chinese, Indonesians, and Singaporeans," would be too much for other Asian groups, such as northern Chinese and Japanese. The experts concluded that the existing WHO BMI cut-off points should be retained as international classifications.

6 "Japanese are not only the longest-lived . . .": Anthony Faiola, "Old, but Not Retiring: Japan's Astoundingly Healthy Seniors," *Washington Post*, October 27, 2004.

6 Data for healthy life expectancy at birth by country are from *World Health Organization World Health Report, 2003* (citing latest figures, as of 2002), available at http://www.who.int/whr/2003/en/Annex4-en.pdf.

7 Table for health care spending contains 2005 estimates from the Economist Intelligence Unit's "Healthcare and Pharmaceuticals Forecast" for the country listed (reports of 2004 and 2005).

8 "Take a stroll through Tokyo . . .": Kelly Baker, "Turning Japanese," *Sunday Mail* (Adelaide), June 22, 2003.

Chapter 1: My Mother's Tokyo Kitchen

11 Epigraph: Donald L. Philippi, *Norito: A Translation of the Ancient Japanese Ritual Prayers* (Princeton, N.J.: Princeton University Press, 1990), p. 82.

19 "Naomi's mother's Tokyo kitchen . . .": Susan D. Plagemann, e-mail to authors.

26 "On the go, I slurped buckwheat noodles . . .": Peggy Orenstein, "Japanese Lessons: What They Know (That We Don't) About Healthy Eating," *Health,* April 2003.

27 For Japanese smoking rates, see "Japan: Food, Beverages and Tobacco Background," Economist Intelligence Unit Executive Briefing, November 11, 2004.

Chapter 2: In a Japanese Tangerine Forest

29 Epigraph: Ota Masayoshi, *Japanese Proverbs* (New York: D.S. Richardson, 1893), p. 11.

30 "a remarkably lovely corner . . ." Jeremy Ferguson, "Festival-Mad Japanese Stage a Fair with a Difference: Expo '94," *The Globe and Mail* (Toronto), August 13, 1994.

31 "The sudden freshness of Japanese cuisine . . .": Donald Richie, *The Donald Richie Reader: Fifty Years of Writing on Japan* (Berkeley, Calif: Stone Bridge Press, 2001), p. 177.

Chapter 3: Seven Secrets from My Mother's Tokyo Kitchen

38 A study of two hundred elderly Japanese women: Greg McKenzie, *Sun Herald* (Australia), July 28, 2002.

39 "When you look at it . . .": Michael A. Lev, "Low-Fat Diet Has Japanese Staying Trim," *Dallas Morning News*, March 30, 1997.

40 Table on daily calorie intakes by country is based on United Nations Food and Agriculture Organization data for 2002, published in *Japan 2005: An International Comparison* (Tokyo: Keizai Koho Center/Japan Institute for Social and Economic Affairs, 2004).

47 "highly aesthetic . . . Various . . ." Bruno Taut is quoted in

Yoshio Tsuchiya, *A Feast for the Eyes: the Japanese Art of Food Arrangement*, trans. Juliet Winters Carpenter (New York: Kodansha, 1985), p. 13.

48 "the importance of 'empty' space . . .": Ibid., p. 37.

51 "Dashi provides Japanese cuisine . . .": Shizuo Tsuji, *Japanese Cooking: A Simple Art* (New York: Kodansha, 1980), p. 146.

51 "a beguiling fragrance . . .": Mark Bittman, "Warmer-Up from Japan," *New York Times,* February 20, 2002.

56 "In Japan, breakfast is the most important . . .": Lisa M. Jensen, "Healthy at 100: Okinawan Diet, Lifestyle May Be Keys to Longevity," *Grand Rapids Press* (Mich.), March 10, 2002.

58 confectionary products per capita: "Japan: Food, Beverages and Tobacco Forecast," Economist Intelligence Unit, June 9, 2005.

60 researchers at Brigham Young University study: BYU press release, "Why We Eat May Be as Important as What We Eat, Say BYU Researchers," June 3, 2003, available at http://byunews.byu.edu/archive03-Jun-usobesity.aspx.

62 "The Japanese are in good health . . .": "How to Live to Be 100," *Time,* August 30, 2004.

63 "As opposed to America . . .": Ibid.

64 "Older Japanese are remarkably healthy . . .": Anthony Faiola, "Old, but Not Retiring: Japan's Astoundingly Healthy Seniors," *Washington Post,* October 27, 2004.

66 "Exercise can cut the risk . . .": Peta Bee, "The Joy of Walking," *The Express* (London), August 24, 2004.

66 David Bassett and Melissa Johnson spoke about 10,000 steps on *Morning Edition*, National Public Radio, May 16, 2005.

85 "It has been said of Japanese food . . .": Junichiro Tanizaki, *In Praise of Shadows*, trans. Thomas J. Harper and Edward G. Seidensticker (London: Jonathan Cape, 1991), pp. 28-29.

Chapter 4: How to Start Your Tokyo Kitchen

94 "is perhaps the single most versatile vegetable . . .": Elizabeth
Andoh, *An American Taste of Japan* (New York: William
Morrow, 1985), p. 23.

Chapter 5: The Seven Pillars of Japanese Home Cooking

123 Epigraph: "If you have . . .": Esther Fisher, "Graceful Art of
Entertaining, Japanese-Style," *The Globe and Mail* (Toronto),
December 28, 1983.

123 Epigraph: "Better than a feast elsewhere . . .": Nina Shire
Ragle, *Even Monkeys Fall from Trees: John Naka's Collection of
Japanese Proverbs* (Laguna Beach, Calif.: Nippon Art Forms,
1987), p. 146.

124 For Queen Himiko and her kingdom, see Delmer M. Brown,
ed., *The Cambridge History of Japan*, vol. 1, *Ancient Japan*
(Cambridge: Cambridge University Press, 1993), pp. 24-29,
287-97, 332-34.

125 Japanese food scholar Hisao Nagayama: Hisao Nagayama,
"Himiko, Ono-no-komachi, Tokugawa Ieyasu Meals," *Brutus*
magazine (Tokyo), October 1, 1988.

125 Schoolchildren honoring Himiko, see "Joyo City Children
Enjoy Himiko Lunch," *Kyoto Shimbun*, January 25, 2005.

127 1692 food guide books: Engelbert Kaempfer, *The History of
Japan, Together with a Description of the Kingdom of Siam, 1690-
92*, trans. J. G. Scheuchzer (Glasgow: J. MacLehose and Sons,
1906), vol. 2, p. 329.

131 "the inner market aisles are clogged . . .": Theodore Bestor,
"Tsukiji, Tokyo's Pantry," *Japan Quarterly*, January 1, 2001.

133 Japan consumes nearly 10 percent of the world's fish: Alex
Renton, "One in Ten Fish Is Eaten in Japan," *The Observer
Food Monthly* (London), April 10, 2005.

133 "Dozens of studies have found . . .": *Harvard Health Letter,* August 1, 2003.

134 "One of the most intriguing . . .": "Omega 3 Fatty Acids," *Heart Disease Weekly*, July 24, 2005.

134 "If you really want to do something . . .": "Fish Provide the Good Oil for Stressed Executives," *National Business Review,* August 23, 2002.

136 For details on fish safety, see the Web site of the Environmental Defense Fund's Oceans Alive project, http://www. oceansalive.org/.

149 Japanese mothers were asked in a poll: Ehara Ayako, "School Meals and Japan's Changing Diet," *Japan Echo,* August 1, 1999.

152 "If you want to say it looks yucky . . .": Peter Landers and Davina Wright, "Seaweed Gets a Place at Table," *The Wall Street Journal*, June 11, 2002.

152 "Rich seaweed tresses . . .": Lady Murasaki, *The Tale of Genji,* trans. Royall Tyler (New York, Viking, 2001), vol. 1, p. 169.

154 "Never in the history of nutrition research . . .": Bradley J. Willcox, D. Craig Willcox, and Makoto Suzuki, *The Okinawa Progam: How the World's Longest-Lived People Achieve Everlasting Health—and How You Can Too* (New York, Three Rivers Press, 2001), p. 74.

155 "The one variable on which . . .:" Loren Cordain and James H. O'Keefe Jr., "Cardiovascular Disease Resulting from a Diet and Lifestyle at Odds with Our Paleolithic Genome: How to Become a 21st-Century Hunter-Gatherer," *Mayo Clinic Proceedings*, January 2004.

156 The five Zen food reflections are from Soei Yoneda with Koei Hoshino and Kim Schuefftan, *The Heart of Zen Cuisine* (Tokyo and New York: Kodansha, 1987), pp. 37, 38.

169 "For the Japanese": Amanda Mayer Stinchecum, "Japanese Rice in Its Many Guises," *New York Times,* March 25, 1990.

170 "And above all there is rice . . .": Junichiro Tanizaki, *In Praise*

of Shadows, trans. Thomas J. Harper and Edward G. Seidensticker (London: Jonathan Cape, 1991), p. 29.

172 "The Japanese believe that pounding rice . . .": Victoria Abbott Riccardi, *Untangling My Chopsticks: A Culinary Sojurn in Kyoto* (New York: Broadway Books, 2003), p. 148.

173 "Long term, the studies show . . .": Jane Snow, "Carbs a Must, Diet Guide Confirms," *South China Morning Post,* February 28, 2005.

174 60 percent of their daily calories from carbohydrates: Ron Bailey, "U.S. Hot Topics: What Is the Japanese Perspective?" *Nutraceuticals World*, July 1, 2004.

186 "soybeans are unique . . .": "Nutrition—What We Still Don't Know About Soy," *Harvard Women's Health Watch*, August 1, 2001.

187 "There have been no double-blind . . .": Laurie Tarkan, "As a Substitute for Hormones, Soy Is Ever More Popular, but Is It Safe?" *New York Times*, August 24, 2004.

187 "soy foods are great . . .": Ibid.

187 "soy foods are best viewed . . .": "Nutrition—What We Still Don't Know About Soy."

187 Dr. George L. Blackburn: Ibid.

194 For Junichiro Koizumi and the astronaut, our sources were the prime minister's Web site, http://www.kantei.go.jp (video clip, accessed August 4, 2005); and Reuters, August 4, 2005.

196 "It's almost like a dream": "Ramen Flying High as Astronaut Cuisine," *Asahi Shimbum,* July 28, 2005.

197 "Last month I found . . .": Elise Tokumasu, e-mail to authors.

198 Statistics on noodle shops and ramen packets are from Julia Moskin, "Here Comes Ramen, the Slurp Heard Round the World," *New York Times,* November 10, 2004.

198 "From documentary evidence": Naomichi Ishige, *The History and Culture of Japanese Food* (London: Kegan Paul, 2001), p. 124.

199 "soba crazy": James Udesky, "The Art of Noodles," *Japan Quarterly,* April 1, 1997.

208 "The tea ceremony requires years . . .": Lafcadio Hearn, *Japan: An Attempt at Interpretation,* (New York: Macmillan, 1904) p. 390.

208 "In my own hands . . .": Bettina Vitell, *The World in a Bowl of Tea* (New York: HarperCollins, 1997), p. vii.

209 "Boil water, infuse tea . . .": Paul Varley and Kumakura Isao, eds., *Tea in Japan: Essays on the History of Chanoyu* (Honolulu: University of Hawaii Press, 1989), p. 4.

209 "When the weather turns warm . . .": Victoria Abbott Riccardi, "Eat Your Tea," *Washington Post,* January 7, 2004.

211 "elixir that creates . . .": Teresa Watanabe "Study Adds to Green Tea's Cancer-Fighting Image," *Chicago Sun-Times,* May 6, 1996.

211 "I believe that there is no Plant . . .": Kaempfer, *The History of Japan,* pp. 240, 241.

212 "impressive activity . . .": Dr. Andrew Weil, *Eating Well for Optimum Health* (New York: Knopf, 2000), p. 139.

212 "We have thousands of years of history . . .": Don Colburn, "Green Tea: Long on History, Short on Facts," *Washington Post,* March 21, 2000.

212 "it's a noncaloric beverage . . .": Ibid.

213 "Meanwhile, let us have a sip . . .": Kakuzo Okakura, *The Book of Tea* (Boston: Shambhala, 2001), p. 14.

216 "It was a lovely summer day . . .": Isabella Bird, *Unbeaten Tracks in Japan* (London: Virago, 1984), p. 138.

219 "It can be conservatively estimated . . .": James J. Gormley, "Just the Fats, Ma'am," *Better Nutrition,* October 1, 1999, citing Walter C. Willett et al, "Trans-fatty Acid Intake in Relation to Risk of Coronary Heart Disease Among Women," *Lancet* 341 (1993): 581-85.

220 "This trans-fatty acid molecule . . .": "Food Industry's Efforts to Help Curb Obesity," *Talk of the Nation,* National Public Radio, July 15, 2003.

220 "very clearly harmful to health . . .": Christopher J. Chipello, "Canada Sets Out to Restrict Trans Fats," *The Wall Street Journal,* December 14, 2004.

221 "Eat more 'good carbs' . . .": "The Atkins Ornish South Beach Zone Diet," *Time,* June 21, 2004.

Chapter 6: The Samurai Diet

231 Epigraph: Scott Bowles, "Hollywood Trades on Interest in Japan," *USA Today*, December 2, 2003.

232 For the story of Tomoe Gozen, her lover, and their battles, see Helen Craig McCullough, trans., *The Tale of the Heike* (Stanford, Calif.: Stanford University Press, 1988), pp. 4-5, 230-93; and Stephen T. Brown, "From Woman Warrior to Peripatetic Entertainer: The Multiple Histories of Tomoe," *Harvard Journal of Asiatic Studies* 58 (June 1998): pp. 183-99.

234 For Nagayama's theory on the role of rice in the Taira-Minamoto clash, see Yu Tani, "Taking Stock—Traditional Japanese Diet—Simply the Best," *Mainichi Daily News* (Tokyo), August 31, 2000.

237 "Even when the shogunate . . .": Stephen Turnbull, *Samurai: The Story of Japan's Great Warriors* (London: PRC Publishing, 2004), p. 130.

238 "They were a kind of mafiosi": Mitsuo Kure, *Samurai: An Illustrated History* (Boston: Tuttle Publishing, 2002), p. 10.

238 "I spurred my horse . . .": Jonathan Norton Leonard and the Editors of Time-Life Books, *Early Japan* (New York: Time-Life Books, 1968), p. 57.

239 "The Asian diet meets every recommendation": Dana Jacobi, "The World's Healthiest Diet, the Asian Diet," *Natural Health*, January 11, 1996.

Another key source for historical background in this chapter is Yoshio Tsuchiya, *A Feast for the Eyes: The Japanese Art of Food Arrangement,* trans. Juliet Winters Carpenter (New York: Kodansha, 1985).

Epilogue: The Great Food Offering

243 The exact details of the imperial great food offering ceremony are shrouded in some mystery, because the ritual is conducted in private. This reconstruction is based on global press coverage of the last such ceremony, held in 1990.

Resources

Japanese Ingredients and Tableware

Many Western supermarkets now carry Japanese foods and ingredients, both in the Asian section and scattered throughout the store. For less common Japanese ingredients, your best source is a local Japanese market or Asian grocery store. Some natural food stores and health food stores carry Japanese items as well.

http://www.ypj.com/en/
To find out if there's a Japanese market near you, go to this "Yellow Pages Japan in USA" English-language Web site, enter the keyword "markets," and then select your city and state.

The following online resources feature Japanese ingredients and Japan-style cookware and tableware.

http://www.amazon.com
http://www.froogle.com
http://shopping.yahoo.com
These shopping portals are good gateways to a wide range of online sources. Search by keywords for the items you need.

http://www.edenfoods.com/store/
One-stop shopping for a variety of essential Japanese home-cooking ingredients, like miso, bonito flakes, udon, and sea vegetables. Click on the "Japanese Traditional" category.

http://www.katagiri.com
Katagiri and Company, Inc.
224 East 59 Street
New York, NY 10022
Tel: 212-755-3566
A food store and online catalog filled with an extensive selection of Japanese ingredients, cookware, and tableware, including hard-to-find items. Not the easiest Web site in the world to navigate, but worth the effort because the selection is very wide. Check out the "Mail Order Catalog" section for both "Japanese Grocery" and "Japanese Gift."

http://www.harney.com/index.html
http://www.itoen.com
For buying Japanese teas online.

Information on Health, Nutrition, Fitness, and Obesity

World Health Organization World Health Report 2005
http://www.who.int/whr/2005/whr2005_en.pdf

International Obesity Task Force
http://www.iotf.org/

USDA MyPyramid, 2005
http://www.mypyramid.gov

U.S. Dietary Guidelines for Americans 2005
http://www.healthierus.gov/dietaryguidelines/

U.S. Government Food and Nutrition Information
http://www.nutrition.gov

Body Mass Index (BMI) calculator
http://www.cdc.gov/nccdphp/dnpa/bmi/calc-bmi.htm

Harvard School of Public Health food pyramids
http://www.hsph.harvard.edu/nutritionsource/pyramids.html

DASH (Dietary Approaches to Stop Hypertension) diet, developed
by the National Heart, Lung and Blood Institute
http://www.nhlbi.nih.gov/health/public/heart/hbp/dash/index.htm

Heart health, obesity, fitness, and related topics
http://www.nhlbi.nih.gov/health/public/heart/index.htm

American Heart Association eating plan for healthy Americans
http://www.americanheart.org/presenter.jhtml?identifier=1088

Fitness and childhood obesity
http://www.shapeup.org/

Seafood safety
http://www.cfsan.fda.gov/seafood1.html
http://www.oceansalive.org/go/seafood

Center for Science in the Public Interest reports
On salmon
http://www.cspinet.org/nah/06_04/farmedsalmon.pdf
On sodium
http://www.cspinet.org/salt/saltreport.pdf

Nutritional composition of specific foods
http://www.nal.usda.gov/fnic/foodcomp/

Health claims on food product labels
http://www.cfsan.fda.gov/~dms/lab-qhc.html

Oldways Preservation Trust (food issues think tank)
http://www.oldwayspt.org/

Japanese Women Don't Get Old or Fat Web site
Visit us at http://www.japanesewomendontgetoldorfat.com

Recipe Index

Acknowledgments

We thank my mother, Chizuko Moriyama, and my father, Shigeo Moriyama, for countless blessings, and especially for sharing their memories, opinions, and family recipes with us.

We thank Mel Berger, our superb agent at William Morris; our terrific editor, Beth Rashbaum; and Irwyn Applebaum, Nita Taublib, Barb Burg, Paulo Pepe, Meghan Keenan, Glen Edelstein, and Kelly Chian at Bantam Dell, as well as our copy editor, Trent Duffy. The acclaimed food writer Victoria Abbott Riccardi was an immense help in advising us on recipes and ingredients.

We are most appreciative to the scientists and doctors who shared their opinions with us, especially Dr. Rudolph E. Tanzi of Harvard Medical School, Professor Tom Kirkwood of the University of Newcastle, Dr. Michel de Lorgeril of the French National Center for Scientific Research, Dr. Antonia Trichopoulou of the University of Athens Medical School, Dr. Laurence Sperling of Emory University School of Medicine, Dr. Robert Vogel of the University of Maryland Medical Center, Professor Jerry Shay of the University of Texas Southwestern Medical Center, Professor Boyd Swinburn of the Australasian Society for the Study of Obesity, Professor Kerin O'Dea of the Menzies School of Health Research in Australia, Professor Roger McCarter of Penn State University, Professor Loren Cordain of Colorado State University, Dr. Walter Bortz of Stanford University Medical School, Dr. Ernst J. Schaefer of the Tufts University School of Medicine, Dr. Lawrence Kushi of Kaiser Permanente, Dr. Toshiie Sakata of the Japanese Society for the Study of Obesity, Dr. Yuji Matsuzawa of Sumitomo Hospital in Osaka, Dr. Yukio Yamori of the International Center for Research on Primary Prevention of Cardiovascular Diseases in Kyoto, Dr. Pedro Kaufmann, Professor Marion Nestle of New York University, Professor Christiaan Leeuwenburgh of the University of Florida College of Medicine, Professor Philip C. Calder of University of Southampton School of Medicine in England, and Dr. Dean Ornish of the Preventive Medicine Research Institute. Institutions are listed for identification purposes.

We thank Mireille Guiliano for writing *French Women Don't Get Fat,* the title of which inspired our own. We also thank Marilou Doyle; Eric Lupfer; Shana Kelly; Raffaella De Angelis; Wayne Furman of the New York Public Library; Shiko Nakamura; Miki, Kazuma, Kasumi, and Ayaka Wako; everyone in the Moriyama and Saito families; Elise Tokumasu; Judy Eldredge; Susan Plagemann; Sara Baer-Sinnott and Birthe Creutz of Oldways Preservation Trust; Joseph and Kate Hooper; Kenji Inadomi; Professor Katarzyna Cwiertka; David Starr; Daniel Rosenblum, Christopher Poston, and Reiko Sassa of the Japan Society in New York; and the staff of the Special Collections Room at the Tokyo Metropolitan Central Library.

Index

About the Authors

NAOMI MORIYAMA was born and raised in Tokyo and spent childhood summers on her grandparents' hillside farm in the Japanese countryside, eating tangerines from the trees and fresh vegetables from the family garden.

She attended college in Illinois, where she gained 25 pounds eating pizza and cookies before moving back to Japan and rediscovering the secrets of her mother Chizuko's Tokyo kitchen.

She moved to New York in her twenties and worked as account executive for Grey Advertising on the Procter & Gamble account and as director of marketing for Home Box Office.

As a U.S.–Japan marketing consultant, she works with some of the world's leading fashion, luxury, and consumer brands and hedge funds.

Three years ago, at the age of forty-two, she was required to display her photo ID at a New York liquor store to prove she was over twenty-one.

Naomi lives in Manhattan with her husband and co-author, William Doyle, and travels to her mother's Tokyo kitchen several times a year. This is her first book.

WILLIAM DOYLE is author of *Inside the Oval Office: The White House Tapes from FDR to Clinton*, a *New York Times* Notable Book of

1999, and *An American Insurrection: James Meredith and the Battle of Oxford, Mississippi, 1962,* which in 2002 won book awards from the American Bar Association and the American Library Association.

In 2004 he co-authored *Dome Raiders: How Scotland Yard Foiled the Greatest Robbery of All Time* with Detective Chief Superintendent Jon Shatford of the London Metropolitan Police. In 1998 he won the Writers Guild of America Award for Best TV Documentary for the A&E special *The Secret White House Tapes,* and he also served as director of original programming for HBO in New York.

He was born in New York and has traveled widely in Japan.